CANCER
CAREGIVING
A TO Z

An At-Home Guide for Patients and Families

CANCER
CAREGIVING
A TO Z

An At-Home Guide for Patients and Families

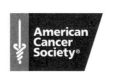

Published by the American Cancer Society/Health Promotions
250 Williams Street NW, Atlanta, GA 30303-1002

Printed in the United States of America

Cover design and composition by Rikki Campbell Ogden/pixiedesign llc

5 4 3 2 1 08 09 10 11 12

Library of Congress Cataloging-in-Publication Data

Cancer caregiving A to Z : an at-home guide for patients and families from the experts at the American Cancer Society.
     p. cm.
  Includes bibliographical references.
  ISBN-13: 978-0-944235-92-8 (pbk.)
  ISBN-10: 0-944235-92-1 (pbk.)
1. Cancer—Patients—Home care—Encyclopedias. 2. Caregivers—Encyclopedias. I. American Cancer Society.

RC266.C338 2008
616.99′4003—dc22
                         2007039969

For more information about cancer, contact your American Cancer Society at **800-ACS-2345** or on the Web at **www.cancer.org**.

Quantity discounts on bulk purchases of this book are available. Book excerpts can also be created to fit specific needs. For information, please contact the American Cancer Society, Health Promotions Publishing, 250 Williams Street NW, Atlanta, GA 30303-1002, or send an e-mail to **trade.sales@cancer.org**.

For special sales, contact us at trade.sales@cancer.org.

A NOTE TO THE READER

The information given here is only a guide; it is not meant to replace talking with your doctor or nurse who know your situation best and can give you the information that you will need the most.

Brand names are used for drugs in this guide because they are sometimes more widely known. The mention of brand names does not represent endorsement by the American Cancer Society. Generic versions or other brand names may be recommended by your doctor or cancer care team.

CONTENTS

INTRODUCTION

When a person is diagnosed with cancer, life changes. But life also changes for the person who helps the patient get through the experience—the caregiver. This person, whether spouse, partner, adult child, or friend, is a valuable participant in the patient's care, and his or her support is crucial to the physical and emotional well-being of the person with cancer.

Today, more people with cancer are being cared for at home. More treatments are done through outpatient or walk-in treatment centers instead of in the hospital. When treatments are done in the hospital, the patient typically spends less time there than in the past. These changes have led to an increase in the involvement of family and friends in the day-to-day care of the person with cancer. Family and friends are taking on responsibilities that, just a short time ago, were reserved for trained health professionals.

A caregiver may take on many roles—from home health aide to companion. A caregiver may help feed, dress, and bathe the patient, as well as arrange schedules, manage insurance issues, and provide transportation. Caregivers serve as legal assistants, financial managers, and housekeepers. They often have to take over the duties the person with cancer once performed, while continuing to meet other family members' needs. In addition, a caregiver can have enormous influence on how the patient deals with his or her illness. The caregiver's encouragement can help the patient stick with a demanding treatment plan and take other steps that are necessary to get well, like eating nutritious meals or getting enough rest.

Cancer Caregiving A to Z provides general information about caring for the person with cancer at home in a simple "a to z" format. This book describes the most common problems associated with cancer, the ways in which problems can be detected early, guidelines for how a caregiver can help with such problems, and the warning signs that indicate a doctor's guidance is needed. This book also lists some of the more common cancer treatments and their possible side effects.

The information presented here is intended to prepare patients and caregivers for some of the problems and concerns they may face. There are also a few suggestions for coping with some of the stresses that come with caring for the person with cancer at home.

Caregivers have an important and unique role to play in helping a loved one through his or her cancer experience. Although caring for someone with cancer can be fulfilling, it can also be demanding and stressful. Communication is helpful in working through tough times, but there is almost always too much for just one person to do. Asking for help or allowing others to help can relieve some of the pressure from caregivers, allowing them also to take care of themselves.

Information, resources, and support for caregivers and patients are available through your local office of the American Cancer Society, on the Web site at **www.cancer.org**, or by calling **800-ACS-2345**, any time, day or night.

Anxiety and Fear

Anxiety is a feeling of worry or unease. Anxiety and fear are common feelings that patients and families sometimes have when coping with cancer. These feelings are normal responses to the stress of the cancer experience and may be noticed more in the first week or two after a cancer diagnosis. Feelings of fear or anxiety may be due to changes in one's ability to continue family duties, loss of control over events in life, changes in appearance or body image, or simply the shock of a cancer diagnosis. These feelings may also stem from uncertainty about the future and concerns about suffering, pain, and the unknown. Fears of loss of independence, changes in relationships with loved ones, and becoming a burden to others may overwhelm the patient and complicate family life.

Family members may feel fear or anxiety because they, too, are uncertain about the future or are angry that their loved one has cancer. They may feel guilty and frustrated that they are not able to "do enough." Or they may feel overwhelmed by everything they now have to do. A caregiver can have stress due to problems with balancing work, child care, self care, and other tasks with more responsibility at home. All of this stress is on top of having to worry about and take care of the person with cancer.

Sometimes a person with cancer becomes overly anxious, fearful, or depressed and may no longer cope well with his or her day-to-day life. If this happens, it often helps the patient and family to seek help from a professional therapist or counselor.

WHAT THE PATIENT CAN DO

▶ Talk about feelings and fears that you or your family members may have. It's okay to feel sad and frustrated.

▶ Decide with your family or caregiver what you can do to support each other.

▶ Avoid blaming yourself and others when you feel anxious and afraid. Instead, try to talk about your feelings and concerns.

▶ Seek help through counseling and support groups. Consider asking your doctor or nurse for a referral to a counselor to work with you and your family.

▶ Use prayer, meditation, or other types of spiritual support.

▶ Try deep breathing and relaxation exercises several times a day. For example, try the following exercise: Close your eyes. Breathe deeply. Concentrate on one body part and relax it, starting with the toes and working up to the head. When you are relaxed, imagine being in a pleasant place, such as a warm beach at sunset or a peaceful meadow.

▶ Cut down on caffeine. It can worsen anxiety symptoms.

▶ Talk with your doctor about the possible use of medicine for anxiety.

WHAT CAREGIVERS CAN DO

▶ Gently invite the patient to talk about his or her fears and concerns. Avoid forcing the patient to talk before he or she is ready.

▶ Listen carefully without judging the patient's feelings— or your own.

▶ Decide with the patient what you can do to support each other.

▶ If the patient is experiencing severe anxiety, reasoning with him or her is usually not helpful. Instead, talk with the doctor about the symptoms and problems you notice.

- Pay attention to your own stress level as well. Try suggestions from the list on the previous page to reduce your own stress, along with any others that have worked for you in the past.

- Consider getting support through groups or individual counseling.

CALL THE DOCTOR if the patient has trouble breathing, is sweating and has a fast or pounding heartbeat, or is more restless than usual.

Note that some medicines or supplements can cause or worsen anxiety symptoms. If anxiety gets worse after the patient begins taking a new medicine, talk with the doctor about it.

For more in-depth information on anxiety and fear, call your American Cancer Society at 800-ACS-2345 and ask for a copy of *Anxiety, Fear, and Depression*. More information is also available on the Web at www.cancer.org.

APPETITE
(POOR OR LOSS OF)

People with a poor appetite or no appetite will eat much less than they normally do or may not eat at all. They may show a lack of interest in food, even refusing to eat favorite foods, and may begin to lose weight. Poor appetite can have a number of causes, such as swallowing problems, anxiety, depression, pain, or nausea and vomiting. It can also be due to a change in sense of taste or smell, feeling full, tumor growth, dehydration, or side effects of chemotherapy or radiation. Poor appetite is most often a short-term problem.

WHAT THE PATIENT CAN DO

- Ask the doctor what may be causing your poor appetite.
- Eat as much as you want, but don't force yourself to eat.
- Think of food as a necessary part of treatment.
- Start the day with breakfast.
- Eat small, frequent meals of your favorite foods.
- Try foods that are high in calories and easy to eat (like pudding, gelatin, ice cream, sherbet, yogurt, and milk shakes).
- Add tasty, high-calorie sauces and gravies to your food, and cut meat into small pieces to make it easier to swallow.
- Use butter, oils, syrups, and milk in foods to raise calories. Avoid low-fat foods unless fats cause heartburn or other problems.
- Try strong flavorings or spices.
- Plan meals that include your favorite foods.

- Create pleasant settings for meals. Soft music, conversation, and other distractions may help you eat more comfortably.
- Eat with other family members.
- Drink liquids between meals instead of with meals. (Liquids at mealtime can lead to early fullness.)
- Try light exercise one hour before meals.
- Hard candies, mint tea, or ginger ale may help get rid of strange tastes in your mouth.
- With your doctor's approval, enjoy a glass of beer or wine before eating.
- Eat a snack at bedtime.
- When you don't feel like eating, try liquid meals of chilled, flavored supplements (such as Ensure, Sustacal, Boost, Carnation Instant Breakfast, and others). Using a straw may help.

WHAT CAREGIVERS CAN DO

- Try giving the patient six to eight small meals and snacks each day.
- Offer starchy foods (like bread, pasta, and potatoes) with high-protein foods (like fish, chicken, meats, turkey, eggs, cheese, milk, tofu, nuts, peanut butter, yogurt, peas, and beans).
- Keep cool drinks and juices within the patient's reach.
- If the smell of food bothers the patient, use the kitchen vent fan to reduce smells. Cover or remove foods with strong or unpleasant smells. You can also serve foods cold or at room temperature, which lessens their smell.
- Create pleasant settings for meals, and eat with the patient.
- Offer fruit smoothies, milk shakes, or liquid meals when the patient doesn't want to eat.
- Try plastic forks and knives instead of metal if the patient is bothered by bitter or metallic tastes.

- Don't blame yourself when the patient refuses food or cannot eat.
- If the patient cannot eat, offer to give him or her a back or foot massage, read aloud, or sit with him or her.

CALL THE DOCTOR if the patient has any of these symptoms:

- Nausea and inability to eat for a day or more
- Weight loss of five pounds or more
- Pain when he or she eats
- No urination for an entire day or no bowel movements for two days or more
- Infrequent urination or urine that comes out in small amounts, is strong-smelling, or is dark in color
- Vomiting for more than twenty-four hours
- Inability to drink or keep down liquids
- Pain that is not controlled

Blood Counts

The term "blood counts" refers to three important parts of your blood: hemoglobin, white blood cells, and platelets. Some cancer treatments can affect these parts of your blood. Your doctor or nurse will monitor your blood counts when you are going through cancer treatment.

The hemoglobin count indicates the ability of the red blood cells to carry oxygen. A normal hemoglobin range is about 14.5 to 18 for men and 12 to 16 for women. Most people still feel well with a hemoglobin level as low as 10. A low hemoglobin level is called anemia.

The white blood cell count measures your body's ability to fight infection. A normal white blood cell count ranges from about 5,000 to 10,000. A low white blood cell count may mean that you are at higher risk of infection. You will want to watch for signs of infection so that you can go to your doctor for treatment right away. A high white blood cell count may be a sign of infection, or it may be due to certain types of disease.

The platelet count looks at the cells that help your blood to clot. A normal platelet count is about 150,000 to 450,000. Normal clotting is still possible with a platelet count of 100,000. Dangerous bleeding may occur when the platelet count goes below 20,000.

It may take a few weeks after cancer treatment for your blood counts to get back to normal. If you see any other doctors or dentists during this time, be sure they know your counts are low. Some very common treatments may cause problems for you. Call the American Cancer Society at 800-ACS-2345 and ask for a copy of *Understanding Your Lab Results* if you would like to know more about what your laboratory results mean. The following sections give more information about low blood counts and what you can do to deal with them.

Low Hemoglobin

A person with low hemoglobin may have new or worsening tiredness that makes it harder to do regular activities. Watch for chest pain or shortness of breath, dizziness, or weakness. Other signs of low hemoglobin include pale skin, nail beds, or gums; vomiting dark brown or bright red material; or bright red, dark red, or black stools (indicating blood in the stool).

WHAT THE PATIENT CAN DO

▶ Balance rest and activities.

▶ Tell the doctor if you're not able to get around as well as usual.

▶ Plan your important activities for times when you have the most energy.

▶ Eat a balanced diet that includes protein (meat, eggs, cheese, and legumes such as peas and beans), and drink eight to ten glasses of water a day, unless your care team gives you other instructions.

WHAT CAREGIVERS CAN DO

▶ Help schedule friends and family members to prepare meals, clean the house, do yard work, or run errands.

▶ Watch for signs of confusion, faintness, or dizziness.

CALL THE DOCTOR if the patient has any of these symptoms:

- Chest pains
- Shortness of breath when resting
- Dizziness or faintness
- Blood in his or her stool
- Confusion or inability to concentrate
- Inability to get out of bed for more than twenty-four hours

Low White Blood Cell Count

A lowered white blood cell count can increase a patient's chance of infection. If the patient has a low number of white blood cells, it is important to watch for signs of infection so that any problems can be treated promptly.

Signs of infection can include a fever of 100.5°F or higher, for temperature taken by mouth; shaking chills (which may be followed by sweating); burning or pain when urinating; sore throat; or sores or white patches in the mouth. Watch also for any new area of redness or swelling, new cough or shortness of breath, or new abdominal pain. Pus or yellowish discharge from an injury or other site is also a sign of infection.

WHAT THE PATIENT CAN DO

▸ Check your temperature by mouth or under the arm if you can't keep a thermometer in your mouth.

▸ If you have fever, take acetaminophen (Tylenol) after calling your doctor. Keep warm.

▸ Take antibiotics or other medicine as prescribed.

▸ Drink two to three quarts of liquid each day, if your doctor approves. However, do not force yourself to drink more than you can tolerate.

▸ Avoid activities that can cause cuts in the skin. If you should get a cut or scrape, wash the injury with soap and water every day, apply antibiotic ointment, and keep it covered until it is healed.

▸ Keep your body clean by bathing daily and washing your hands after using the bathroom.

▸ Avoid crowds and don't visit with people who have infections, coughs, or fevers.

▸ Talk with your doctor or nurse about eating raw fruits and vegetables. Some suggest eating only cooked fruits and vegetables until the white blood cell counts come up again. If you eat raw foods, wash them carefully and peel them to avoid germs.

- Keep your mouth clean by brushing your teeth twice daily and flossing once daily (unless you were told not to floss).

- Use a stool softener to avoid constipation and straining to have a bowel movement. Do not use enemas or suppositories of any kind. If you are constipated, check with your doctor before using laxatives. (See the section on constipation on page 26.)

WHAT CAREGIVERS CAN DO

- Watch for shaking chills. If they occur, check the patient's temperature by mouth or under the arm after the shaking stops. Do not take a rectal temperature.

- Request that visitors who have fevers or any contagious illnesses visit the patient only by phone until they are well.

- Offer the patient extra fluids.

- Help the patient take his or her medicines on schedule.

CALL THE DOCTOR if the patient has any of these symptoms:

- Fever of 100.5°F or higher, for temperature taken by mouth

- Shaking chills

- Feeling or seeming "different" to others

- Inability to take fluids

Low Platelet Count

Platelets help your blood to clot, so a low platelet count can result in bleeding. Watch for bleeding from anywhere (such as the mouth, nose, or rectum); new bruises; a red rash that looks like pinpoint dots (usually starting on the feet and legs); or headaches, dizziness, or blurred vision. Other signs to look for include weakness that gets worse; joint or muscle pain; vomiting blood or dark material that looks like coffee grounds; bright red, dark red, or black stools (indicating blood in the stool); and increased vaginal bleeding during monthly periods.

WHAT THE PATIENT CAN DO

▶ Use only an electric razor (not a blade) for shaving.

▶ Avoid contact sports (such as wrestling, boxing, or football) and any other activities that might result in injury.

▶ Protect your skin from cuts, scrapes, and sharp objects.

▶ Use a soft toothbrush, and talk to your doctor or nurse about whether you should put off flossing your teeth until platelet counts improve. For mouth bleeding, rinse your mouth with cold water.

▶ Do not blow your nose or cough with great force.

▶ Stay upright; keep your head level with or above your heart.

▶ Avoid placing anything in the rectum, including suppositories or thermometers.

▶ Stay away from anti-inflammatory pain medicines, such as naproxen or ibuprofen, or aspirin-containing medicines unless you first clear it with your doctor.

▶ If bleeding starts, stay calm. Sit or lie down and call for help.

WHAT CAREGIVERS CAN DO

▶ For nosebleeds, have the patient sit up with the head tilted forward to keep blood from dripping down the back of the throat. Put ice on the patient's nose and pinch the nostrils shut for five minutes before releasing them. Ice on the back of the neck may also help.

▶ For bleeding from other areas, press on the bleeding area with a clean, dry washcloth until the bleeding stops.

 CALL THE DOCTOR if the patient has any of the symptoms above, or if he or she has trouble moving or speaking.

Blood in Stool

Blood in the stool may occur as a result of irritation of the bowel during a bowel movement. It can also be caused by straining very hard, an ulcer or a tumor in the bowel, hemorrhoids (enlarged blood vessels in or around the anus), a pressure sore or ulcer in the anal area, or a low platelet count. The patient might notice blood on his or her underwear or sheets or blood on toilet paper.

WHAT THE PATIENT CAN DO

▶ Avoid placing anything in your rectum, including suppositories or thermometers.

▶ Keep your stool soft by taking in plenty of fluids and fiber. Use stool softeners, and avoid enemas or laxatives.

▶ Wash your anal area very carefully with warm, soapy water, rinse well, and pat dry.

▶ A sitz bath (sitting in warm water) may be helpful for hemorrhoids.

▶ If you are seeing signs of blood in your stool, monitor the amount and frequency of blood being passed.

WHAT CAREGIVERS CAN DO

▶ Help the patient watch for bleeding.

▶ Offer the patient extra fluids, fruits, and vegetables to keep stools soft.

CALL THE DOCTOR if the patient sees blood on the toilet paper two or more times, or if he or she has streaks of blood in the stool, bright red blood from the rectum, or dark red or black bowel movements. (Note: Eating beets can cause red stools, and iron tablets or bismuth medicines such as Pepto-Bismol and Kaopectate can temporarily cause black stools. This is normal.)

Blood in Urine

Blood can be seen in the urine when a patient is bleeding in some part of the urinary system and the blood is being flushed out along with the urine. Common causes include urinary tract infections (UTIs), kidney or bladder stones, injury to the urinary tract, a tumor growing in the urinary tract, or problems with blood clotting. (See the section on blood counts on page 7.) The patient may notice that his or her urine is red, pink, or tea-colored, or that there is blood or clots in the urine. Urination may be painful.

WHAT THE PATIENT CAN DO

▶ Drink about one quart of water or other fluids during each eight-hour period (three quarts each day), unless your doctor has limited the amount you can drink.

▶ Take your medicines as prescribed.

WHAT CAREGIVERS CAN DO

▶ Offer the patient extra fluids.

▶ Help the patient look for signs of blood in urine, if needed.

CALL THE DOCTOR if the patient has any of these symptoms:

- Blood in the urine or discolored urine
- Pain in lower back or on lower sides of back when urinating
- Pink, cloudy, or foul-smelling urine
- Sudden, urgent need to urinate
- More frequent urination
- Inability to urinate
- Shaking chills or fever of 100.5°F or higher, for temperature taken by mouth
- Confusion or feeling or seeming "different"
- Any urinary symptoms that do not improve after treatment

Bone Marrow or Stem Cell Transplants

Stem cells are cells in the bone marrow (the spongy matter in certain bones) that constantly make blood cells for the body. Stem cell transplants are used to restock the bone marrow with these cells when they have been destroyed by chemotherapy, radiation, or disease. Stem cells can be taken from bone marrow or blood, and they may be the patient's own (called autologous) or may come from someone else (called allogeneic).

Bone marrow transplants were the first method for replacing stem cells, but are used less often today. In this procedure, donors are usually given medicine to make them sleep before bone marrow can be taken for transplant. Your doctor or cancer care team will be able to tell you more about treatment or clinical trials using stem cell transplants.

If the patient has had a bone marrow transplant or stem cell transplant, it is important to be aware of potential problems or side effects so that you can notify the doctor or cancer care team.

WHAT PATIENTS CAN DO

▸ Go to every scheduled appointment and take all medicines exactly as prescribed.

▸ Ask questions and take notes during appointments. Your cancer care team will assist you in answering your questions.

▸ Ask about side effects and what to do if they occur.

▸ Ask when you should notify your doctor of any changes.

WHAT CAREGIVERS CAN DO

▸ Go with the patient to appointments and ask the care team about any concerns you have.

- Help ensure that the patient takes all medicines exactly as prescribed.
- Help watch for and monitor any side effects and symptoms.

CALL THE DOCTOR if you have any questions or concerns or if the patient has any of these symptoms:

- Skin rashes, especially on palms of hands or soles of feet
- Poor appetite and/or weight loss
- Shortness of breath or cough
- Tiredness or fatigue
- Pain or aching
- Stomach cramps
- Nausea or vomiting
- Mouth sores or dryness
- Diarrhea
- Yellowing of the skin or whites of eyes
- Dizziness, paleness, or other signs of low hemoglobin (See page 8 for other signs of low hemoglobin.)
- Fever, shaking chills, or other signs of infection (See page 9 for other signs of infection.)
- Blood in stool or urine, or bleeding from anywhere (See the section on low platelet count on pages 10–11.)

For more in-depth information on bone marrow or stem cell transplants, call your American Cancer Society at 800-ACS-2345 and ask for a copy of *Bone Marrow and Peripheral Blood Stem Cell Transplants*. Information is also available on the Web at www.cancer.org.

CHEMOTHERAPY

Chemotherapy, often called "chemo" for short, is the use of drugs to kill cancer cells. The drugs are most often given intravenously, but some agents may be given in the form of pills or injections. The drugs enter the bloodstream and reach all areas of the body. Chemotherapy may be used along with surgery and other types of treatment in hopes of a cure, a remission or, in advanced cancer, as a means of relieving symptoms.

Chemotherapy drugs may be injected directly into the affected area of the body. This is called regional chemotherapy and is only used for certain types of cancer. It allows a higher dose of medicine to go directly to the cancer site.

Side effects from chemotherapy depend on the type of drug, how much is used, how often it is given, and for how long. Side effects can include short-term hair loss, fatigue, nausea, and vomiting. Drugs and other treatments can help with the side effects of chemotherapy. Many patients have few or no side effects, and you may be among those who have few problems. No one can predict who will and will not have them.

WHAT THE PATIENT CAN DO

▶ Find out what chemotherapy drugs you will be taking, how they will be given, and how often and how long you will get them.

▶ Ask your doctor or nurse about side effects that might happen with the drugs you are taking and what you can do to prevent or reduce them.

▶ Ask about activities you should or should not do during chemotherapy.

- Talk with your doctor about how chemotherapy will affect your plans to have children. (See the section on sexuality on page 96 for more information.)
- Do not get pregnant while you are getting chemotherapy. Ask your doctor how long you should wait after chemotherapy to try to get pregnant.
- Learn how to contact your doctor or nurse during non-office hours.
- Find out whether you should take vitamins or supplements during your chemotherapy.
- Before chemotherapy starts, get all your prescriptions filled and be sure you understand how to use each one.
- Go to every scheduled appointment.
- Once you have begun chemotherapy, report all side effects to your doctor.

This book includes information on many of the possible side effects that can happen when you are undergoing chemotherapy, such as fever, fatigue, hair loss, mouth sores, and nausea and vomiting. If you have questions or are experiencing any side effects, speak to your doctor and see the relevant sections in this book for more information.

WHAT CAREGIVERS CAN DO

- Go with the patient to appointments, especially on chemotherapy days.
- If you are unable to drive or go for appointments, talk with the social worker or nurse at the doctor's office to get help.
- Know how to get in touch with the patient's doctor, even when the office is closed.
- If the patient is unable to go to an appointment, talk with the doctor or nurse as soon as possible and plan what to do next.

- Be sure that someone is with the patient during the first couple of days after each chemotherapy treatment, since he or she may need more help at those times.

- Help watch for side effects and symptoms.

> **CALL THE DOCTOR** if the patient has any of these symptoms:
>
> - Any side effect that lasts more than one day
> - Fever of 100.5°F or higher, for temperature taken by mouth
> - Any bleeding
> - Pain or redness at the site where the chemotherapy was administered

For more in-depth information on chemotherapy, call the American Cancer Society at 800-ACS-2345 and ask for a copy of *Understanding Chemotherapy: A Guide for Patients and Families*, or find more information on the Web at www.cancer.org. You can also get information on the specific chemotherapy drug(s) you will be taking.

CLINICAL TRIALS

Before a new treatment can be used on people, researchers study it in a laboratory. If laboratory studies suggest the treatment will work, the next step is to test its value for patients. These studies in humans are called clinical trials. Clinical trials are needed to find new and better ways to treat people with cancer. You cannot be placed in a clinical trial without volunteering for it, being informed about it, and signing a special consent form.

Through clinical trials, researchers try to answer several questions:

▶ Does this treatment work?

▶ Does it work better than treatments currently in use?

▶ What side effects does it cause?

▶ Do the benefits outweigh the risks?

▶ What patients are most likely to find this treatment helpful?

During your treatment, your doctor may suggest that you think about a clinical trial. This does not mean that you are being asked to serve as a human "guinea pig." Nor does it mean that your case is hopeless and that your doctor is suggesting a last-ditch effort. A clinical trial is done only when there is some reason to believe that the treatment being studied may be more helpful than what is now in use.

Ask your doctor if there is a clinical trial that might be right for you. Then learn all you can about it. There may be risks as well as benefits. If you change your mind after enrolling in a clinical trial, you can still leave the trial at any time.

▸ Ask questions. Here are some of the questions you can ask when deciding whether a clinical trial is right for you:

- What is the purpose of the clinical trial?

- What does the clinical trial involve? What kinds of tests and treatments are part of the trial?

- Are there other treatments that might work for me if I do not take part in the clinical trial?

- How will the study affect my daily life?

- What side effects might result from the treatment? What can I do about them?

- How long will the study last?

- Will I need to be in the hospital? For how long and how often?

- How much does the treatment cost? Will any of it be free? If costs are incurred, will my insurance cover them?

- If I'm harmed as a result of the clinical trial, what kind of treatment would be offered?

- What type of long-term follow-up care is offered as part of the clinical trial?

- What will happen if I decide to drop out of the clinical trial?

WHAT CAREGIVERS CAN DO

▸ Encourage the patient to ask the doctor about clinical trials.

▸ Go with the patient to learn about any clinical trial he or she is considering.

▸ Be sure the patient's questions have been answered to his or her satisfaction before enrolling in a clinical trial.

For more in-depth information on clinical trials, call your American Cancer Society at 800-ACS-2345 and ask for a copy of *Clinical Trials: What You Need to Know*. More information is also available on the Web at www.cancer.org.

Confusion

If a person has trouble thinking and acting as he or she normally does, or if his or her thought process seems to be disturbed, the person may be confused. Confusion can be caused by a number of things, including low blood sugar, infection, high fever, tumor spread into the brain, cancer in the fluid surrounding the brain, lack of oxygen to the brain, too much calcium in the blood, intense pain, or too much pain medicine. Confusion can begin or worsen when the patient is in a new place and may worsen at night. Usually, doctors can and should treat the cause of the confusion.

A patient who has become confused may experience a sudden change in the ability to speak, marked especially by long pauses or slurred words. The patient may have trouble staying alert or paying attention, and may forget what he or she is doing. Other signs of confusion include sudden changes in emotion; cloudy, disorganized thinking or not knowing where he or she is; and a change in the person's ability to bathe and dress when it was manageable before. If a person becomes confused, call the doctor right away. The patient may need to see the doctor quickly so that the doctor can find and treat the cause of the problem. Sometimes the patient may need to be in the hospital while the problem is being treated.

WHAT THE PATIENT CAN DO

- ▶ Call the doctor right away if you realize you are having periods of confusion.
- ▶ Ask someone to stay with you to help keep you safe.

WHAT CAREGIVERS CAN DO

▶ Go to doctor's appointments with the patient so that you can describe the patient's problems and remember instructions for him or her.

▶ When talking to the patient, talk slowly and use short sentences. Stay within a few feet of the patient, and turn off the radio or television when you are talking. You might also try to focus the patient's attention by gently touching the patient and facing him or her. Always tell the patient who you are.

▶ Remind the patient of the day, time, and where he or she is. It can help to keep a calendar and clock where the patient can see them.

▶ Tell the patient just before you start doing something (such as changing the bed, dressing them, or bathing them), and explain each step as you go along.

▶ Play soft, soothing music when the patient is in the room alone.

▶ Use a night light so that the patient can see where he or she is.

▶ Label commonly used items with pictures indicating their purpose. For example, put a picture of a toilet on the bathroom door and a picture of a flame over the stove.

▶ Protect the patient from injury. For example, use side rails if the patient might get out of bed and not know where he or she is. Help the patient with washing, going to the bathroom, and other daily activities that may be hard for him or her to do alone.

▶ Keep track of what the patient eats. He or she may forget to eat or may be unable to eat without assistance.

▶ Be sure that the patient takes the right medicines as prescribed, and keep medicines out of reach between doses.

CALL THE DOCTOR if the patient has any of these symptoms:

- Sudden confusion or confusion that worsens
- Sudden changes in the ability to do routine tasks or care for oneself
- Violent behavior
- Self-inflicted harm

CONSTIPATION

Constipation is the infrequent or difficult passage of hard feces (stool), which often causes pain and discomfort. It is caused by too little fluid or not enough movement in the bowel. Lack of activity, weakness, ignoring the urge to have a bowel movement, pain medicine, or poor food and fluid intake can all add to this problem. A patient with constipation may have small, hard bowel movements, stomachache or cramps, feelings of fullness or discomfort, and frequent gas or belching. Constipation can be accompanied by nausea or vomiting, a swollen or puffy-appearing belly, or the leakage of soft stool that looks like diarrhea.

WHAT THE PATIENT CAN DO

▶ Drink more fluids. Pasteurized fruit juices and warm or hot fluids in the morning are especially helpful.

▶ Increase the amount of fiber in the daily diet by eating foods like whole grain breads and cereals; fresh raw fruits with skins; fresh raw vegetables; fruit juices; and dates, apricots, raisins, prunes, prune juice, and nuts.

▶ Avoid foods and drinks that cause gas, such as cabbage, broccoli, and carbonated drinks.

▶ Try to avoid any foods that can cause constipation, such as cheese or eggs.

▶ Get as much light exercise as you can.

▶ Do not use enemas or suppositories. Use stool softeners or laxatives only after talking with your doctor or nurse.

▶ Go to the bathroom as soon as you have the urge to have a bowel movement.

▶ Keep a record of your bowel movements so that problems can be noticed quickly.

▸ Offer the patient prune juice, hot lemon water, or tea to help stimulate bowel movements.

▸ Encourage the patient to drink extra fluids.

▸ Help keep a record of the patient's bowel movements.

▸ Offer high-fiber foods such as whole grains, dried fruits, and bran.

▸ Talk with the doctor before giving the patient laxatives.

CALL THE DOCTOR if the patient has any of these symptoms:

• No bowel movement in forty-eight hours

• Blood in or around the anal area or in stool (See page 12 for information on blood in the stool.)

• Inability to move bowels within one or two days after taking a laxative

• Cramps or vomiting that won't stop

• Constipation for several days, followed by small amounts of diarrhea or oozing of liquid stool, which could suggest an impaction (severe constipation)

DEPRESSION

Some degree of depression is common when patients and family members are coping with cancer. Sadness and grief are normal and part of the range of emotions. But when these feelings last a long time or get in the way of day-to-day activities, there is reason for concern. Clinical depression, a treatable illness, occurs in about twenty-five percent of people with cancer. Depression causes distress, impaired functioning, and a lowered ability to follow treatment plans. People who have had one or more bouts of serious depression are more likely to have depression after their cancer diagnosis.

It is not unusual for patients to have symptoms of anxiety and depression at the same time. (See page 1 for more on fear and anxiety.) Family and friends can help by watching for symptoms of depression in a cancer patient and encouraging him or her to seek help if necessary. Treatments for depression include medication, counseling, or a combination of both, and sometimes other specialized treatments. These treatments can alleviate depression, reduce suffering, and help the patient have a better quality of life.

These are the symptoms of clinical depression:

▸ Sad or "empty" mood almost every day for most of the day

▸ Loss of interest or pleasure in activities that were once enjoyed

▸ Eating problems (loss of appetite or overeating), including weight loss or gain

▸ Sleep changes (inability to sleep, early waking, or oversleeping)

▸ Decreased energy or fatigue almost every day

▸ Feelings of guilt, worthlessness, and helplessness

- Trouble concentrating, remembering, or making decisions
- Thoughts of death or suicide or suicide attempts
- Wide mood swings from depression to periods of agitation and high energy
- Restless or "slowed down" behavior almost every day

If five or more of these symptoms last for two weeks or longer, or are severe enough to hinder normal functioning, an evaluation for clinical depression by a qualified health or mental health professional is recommended.

WHAT THE PATIENT CAN DO

- Talk about the feelings and fears that you or your family members may have. It's okay to feel sad and frustrated.
- Listen carefully to each other, encouraging each other to talk, but not forcing the issue.
- Decide together what you can do to support each other.
- Seek help through counseling and support groups. Consider working with a professional counselor to deal with the changes in your life. Some people are also helped by prayer or other types of spiritual support.
- Try deep breathing and relaxation exercises several times a day. For example, try this exercise: Close your eyes. Breathe deeply. Concentrate on each body part and relax it, starting with your toes and working up to your head. When you are relaxed, imagine being in a pleasant place, such as a breezy beach or a sunny meadow.
- Talk with your doctor about possible treatments for anxiety or depression. Be sure the doctor has a list of all drugs you are taking before antidepressants are started.
- If you begin taking antidepressants, expect to wait at least two to four weeks for depression to improve. Continue to take all your medicines as prescribed. Sometimes stimulant drugs are used during this time to relieve symptoms.
- Let your doctor know if you are having side effects after starting an antidepressant.

- Avoid alcohol while on an antidepressant unless approved by your doctor or pharmacist.
- Find out if the antidepressant causes drowsiness before you try to drive.
- Do not suddenly stop taking the antidepressant medicine.

WHAT CAREGIVERS CAN DO

- Gently invite the patient to talk about his or her fears and concerns. Avoid forcing the patient to talk before he or she is ready.
- Listen carefully without judging the patient's feelings—or your own. It is okay to point out and disagree with negative or self-defeating thoughts.
- Decide together what you can do to support each other.
- Avoid telling the person to "cheer up" if he or she is depressed.
- Do not try to reason with the person if fear, anxiety, or depression is severe. Talk with the doctor about medicines and other kinds of help.
- If necessary, help make the appointment for evaluation or treatment and take the patient to the doctor.
- If the patient starts antidepressants, encourage him or her to continue treatment until symptoms are improved (usually two to four weeks) or to seek different treatment if symptoms don't improve.
- Reassure the patient that with time and treatment, he or she will begin to feel better.
- Engage the person in activities he or she enjoys.

Keep in mind that caregivers can also become depressed. All of the suggestions above apply to caregivers, too. Take time to care for yourself. Spend time with friends or doing activities you enjoy. Consider getting support for yourself through groups or individual counseling.

CALL THE DOCTOR if the patient has any of these symptoms:

- Thoughts of suicide or constant thoughts about death

- Behavior that provokes concern for his or her safety

- Inability to eat or sleep and lack of interest in activities of daily living for several days

- Trouble breathing, sweating, or restlessness

For more in-depth information on depression, call your American Cancer Society at 800-ACS-2345 and ask for a copy of *Anxiety, Fear, and Depression*. More information is also available on the Web at www.cancer.org.

Diarrhea

Diarrhea is the passage of loose or watery stools three or more times a day with or without discomfort. It happens when water in the intestine is not absorbed back into the body. Sometimes diarrhea can be caused by an overflow of intestinal liquids around stool that is lodged in the intestine (a condition called impaction). Other causes can include infections; surgery; anxiety; side effects of chemotherapy, radiation therapy to the abdomen, or medicines; supplemental feedings containing large amounts of vitamins, minerals, sugar, and electrolytes; and tumor growth. Diarrhea caused by chemotherapy or radiation therapy may last for up to three weeks after treatment ends.

WHAT THE PATIENT CAN DO

▸ Try a clear liquid diet (including items like water, weak tea, apple juice, peach nectar, clear broth, frozen ice pops, and plain gelatin) as soon as diarrhea starts or when you feel that it's going to start. Avoid acidic drinks such as tomato juice, citrus juices, and fizzy soft drinks.

▸ Eat frequent small meals. Do not eat foods that are very hot or spicy.

▸ Avoid greasy foods, bran, raw fruits and vegetables, and caffeine.

▸ Avoid pastries, candies, rich desserts, jellies, preserves, and nuts.

▸ Do not drink alcohol or use tobacco.

▸ Avoid milk and milk products if they seem to make your diarrhea worse.

- Be sure your diet includes foods that are high in potassium (bananas, potatoes, apricots, and sports drinks such as Gatorade or Powerade). Potassium is an important mineral that you may lose if you have diarrhea.

- Monitor the amount and frequency of your bowel movements.

- After each bowel movement, clean your anal area with a mild soap, rinse well with warm water, and pat dry. Sitting in a tub of warm water or a sitz bath can help reduce discomfort.

- Apply a water-repellent ointment, such as A&D Ointment or petroleum jelly, to the anal area.

- Take medicine for diarrhea as directed by your doctor. Be sure to check with the doctor before using any over-the-counter diarrhea medicine. Many of these contain compounds that can worsen bleeding problems. It may be more appropriate to use a prescription medicine.

- When the diarrhea starts to improve, try eating small amounts of foods that are easy to digest, such as rice, bananas, applesauce, yogurt, mashed potatoes, low-fat cottage cheese, and dry toast, for a day or two. If diarrhea continues to improve, start small, regular meals.

WHAT CAREGIVERS CAN DO

- See that the patient drinks about three quarts of fluids each day.

- Keep a record of the patient's bowel movements to help decide when the doctor should be called.

- Check the anal area for red, scaly, broken skin. If this is present, consult the doctor.

- Protect the bed and chairs from being soiled by putting pads with plastic backing under the buttocks where the patient will lie down or sit.

CALL THE DOCTOR if the patient has any of these symptoms:

- Six or more loose bowel movements per day with no improvement in two days

- Blood in or around the anal area or in the stool (See page 12 for more about blood in stool.)

- Weight loss of five or more pounds after diarrhea starts

- New abdominal pain or cramps for two days or more

- No urination for twelve hours or more

- Inability to drink liquids for forty-eight hours or more

- Fever of 100.5°F or higher, for temperature taken by mouth

- A puffy or swollen belly

- Constipation for several days, followed by small amounts of diarrhea or oozing of liquid stool, which could suggest an impaction (severe constipation)

DIFFICULTY MOVING

The patient may have general weakness and problems walking and may find it hard to get from one place to another. When a person spends a lot of time in bed, muscles become weaker. Other things that can make it hard to move include pain in the joints or legs or some of the side effects of chemotherapy and radiation. It is important to move and exercise as much as possible to prevent new problems. Problems caused by a lower level of activity may include loss of appetite, constipation, skin sores, difficulty breathing, stiff joints, and mental changes.

WHAT THE PATIENT CAN DO

▸ Do active or passive range-of-motion exercises as instructed by the nurse, doctor, or physical therapist. (See page 37 for more on exercise.)

▸ Take your pain medicines as prescribed.

▸ Drink as much liquid as allowed by your doctor.

▸ Keep a record of your bowel movements, and follow the recommendations on page 26 to reduce the risk of constipation.

▸ When in bed, turn and change positions at least every two hours.

▸ When walking or standing, wear shoes (not slippers that slide off easily). Use any brace, cane, walker, or other support prescribed by your doctor or nurse.

▸ Take short walks if you can. Even if you are bedridden, try to sit up in a chair for meals and walk to the bathroom or bedside commode.

▸ If you need help when walking, have a family member support you on your weakest side.

▸ When lifting the patient, keep your back straight and bend and lift from your knees and hips. Stand as close to the patient as possible, and keep your feet spread for a firm base and good balance.

▸ If the patient needs help walking, you can help by supporting the patient on his or her weakest side. For example, if the right side is weak, stand on that side before he or she gets up. Put your left arm around the patient and put his or her right forearm and hand in front of your right shoulder.

▸ Always lock the wheels on the bed or wheelchair.

▸ Always pull the patient toward you when rolling him or her in bed.

▸ Clear the floor of any hazards so that you can help the person to a chair or to the bathroom without tripping over rugs, cords, fallen objects, or clothing or slipping on liquids.

▸ If the patient is unsteady but still able to get up, it is important to take precautions so the patient doesn't fall. See pages 39–40 for more on preventing falls.

▸ If the patient is to be alone for awhile, be sure that the phone and emergency phone numbers are within easy reach.

▸ As instructed by the nurse, doctor, or physical therapist, do passive range-of-motion exercises with the patient.

CALL THE DOCTOR if the patient has any of these symptoms:

- Increasing weakness
- Falls
- Headache, blurred vision, numbness, or tingling
- Change in mental status, like getting confused, disoriented, or very sleepy
- Pain that gets worse

EXERCISE

It is important to exercise as much as you can to keep muscles working as well as possible. Exercise helps prevent problems that are caused by long-term bed rest, such as stiff joints, weak muscles, breathing problems, constipation, skin sores, poor appetite, and mental changes. It also helps reduce stress and relieve fatigue. Talk with your doctor about exercises that you can do safely, and then set goals for gradually increasing your physical activity level. If you have trouble moving around, see page 35.

WHAT THE PATIENT CAN DO

▸ Do as much daily self-care as possible.

▸ Take a walk every day.

▸ Do range-of-motion exercises as instructed by your nurse, doctor, or physical therapist. Active range-of-motion exercises are when you move a joint without any help from others. Passive range-of-motion exercises are when someone else moves it for you. If needed, you can do these exercises without getting out of bed. Avoid moving any joint that is painful.

WHAT CAREGIVERS CAN DO

▸ Go with the patient on walks or other exercise outings.

▸ Encourage the patient to do as much as possible for himself or herself.

▸ Talk with the doctor or nurse about range-of-motion exercises if the patient has trouble getting out of bed. Remind the patient to do active range-of-motion exercises several times a day, if he or she is able. If not, you may learn to help the patient with passive range-of-motion exercises.

CALL THE DOCTOR if the patient has any of these symptoms:

- Weakness, loss of balance, or falls
- New pain or pain that gets worse
- Headaches or dizziness
- Blurred vision, new numbness, or tingling in arms or legs

FALLS

A person who is unsteady on his or her feet, confused, or weak is at high risk for falling. Some of the most common situations in which falls occur include trying to get out of bed, falling off the toilet, slipping in the bathtub or shower, or tiring out and falling while walking.

WHAT THE PATIENT CAN DO

▸ If you feel weak or your balance feels "off," ask for help getting up or walking. Before you get up, sit on the side of the bed for a minute or so. This may help if the change in position causes dizziness.

▸ If you fall, let your doctor and your caregivers know. They will want to help prevent future falls and may need to check you for injuries.

▸ If you are having trouble walking, ask your doctor about a home health care nursing visit. Home health care nurses may be able to make your home safer for you. They also have ways to help you walk more safely.

WHAT CAREGIVERS CAN DO

▸ When the patient needs to get out of bed, have him or her sit on the side of the bed for a minute or so. This will help if the change in position causes the patient to be dizzy or unsteady.

▸ If the patient is unsteady, help support him or her.

▸ If the patient feels light-headed, stay with the patient when he or she goes to the bathroom.

▸ Use side rails on the patient's bed.

▸ Put bath mats or nonslip stickers in the tub or shower. You can also use a shower stool or chair so the patient can sit while bathing.

- Keep electrical cords off the floor and tape edges of rugs to the floor. Walking paths need to be clear of clothing, throw rugs, and other items that can cause tripping or slipping.

- Have a bedpan or urinal within easy reach. If possible, place a commode near the bed or place the bed near the bathroom.

- The patient should wear shoes or nonskid slippers when walking or standing. Avoid using slippery shoes or open-heeled bedroom slippers.

- Ask the doctor about a home health care visit to check your home for ways to prevent falls. Handrails, bedside commodes, grab bars, shower chairs, and other tools can help some patients to move about their home more easily.

CALL THE DOCTOR if the patient has any of these symptoms:

- New weakness or numbness
- Confusion or disorientation
- Forgetfulness
- Isn't making sense
- Unsteadiness to the point that a fall is likely

If the patient falls, follow these suggestions:

- Leave the patient where he or she has fallen until you can find out if there are serious injuries.

- If the patient is unconscious, bleeding, or has fluid draining from the mouth, ears, or nose, call the doctor or 911 right away.

- If the patient is not breathing, call 911 unless the patient is in hospice or has a durable power of attorney for health care that states his or her wish not to be revived.

- If the patient is conscious, ask if he or she feels any pain.

- Check the patient's head, arms, legs, and buttocks for cuts and bruises, and to see if anything looks strange or misshapen (possibly due to a broken bone).
- Apply ice packs and pressure to any bleeding area. (Put ice in a plastic bag and wrap bag in a towel.)
- If you cannot move the patient, make him or her as comfortable as possible until help comes.
- If the patient is not in pain and is not bleeding, help him or her back to bed or to a chair. If possible, have two people move the patient.

FATIGUE

Fatigue is when a person has less energy to do the things he or she normally does or wants to do. Fatigue is the most common side effect of cancer treatment. This is different from the tiredness that comes with everyday life. Fatigue related to cancer treatment can appear suddenly and can be overwhelming. It is not relieved by rest. It can last for months after treatment ends. This type of fatigue can affect many aspects of a person's life, including the ability and desire to do usual activities. Patients suffering from fatigue may have no energy, sleep more, and still feel tired even after rest. They may give less attention to their personal appearance and can have trouble thinking, concentrating, and remembering words.

Cancer fatigue is real and should not be ignored. It can be worse when a person is dehydrated, anemic, in pain, not sleeping well, or has an infection. (See the related sections in this book for more information about these issues.) Recent studies have shown that exercise programs during treatment can help reduce fatigue.

WHAT THE PATIENT CAN DO

▸ Balance rest and activities.

▸ Tell the doctor if you're not able to get around as well as usual.

▸ Plan your important activities for when you have the most energy.

▸ Schedule necessary activities throughout the day rather than all at once.

▸ Get enough rest and sleep. Short naps and rest breaks may be needed.

- Ask others to help you by cooking meals and doing housework, yard work, and errands.

- Eat a balanced diet that includes protein (meat, eggs, cheese, and legumes such as peas and beans) and drink about eight to ten glasses of water a day, unless your cancer care team gives you other instructions.

- Exercise can help reduce fatigue. See page 37 for more on exercise.

- Remember that fatigue caused by cancer treatment is a short-term problem. Your energy will slowly get better after treatment has ended.

WHAT CAREGIVERS CAN DO

- Help schedule friends and family members to prepare meals, clean the house, do yard work, or run errands for the patient.

- Try not to push the patient to do more than he or she is able.

- Help the patient set up a routine for activities during the day.

CALL THE DOCTOR if the patient has any of these symptoms:

- Tiredness that prevents getting out of bed for more than a twenty-four-hour period

- Confusion or inability to think clearly

- Trouble sleeping at night

- Fatigue that keeps getting worse

- Shortness of breath or racing heart after just a little activity

FEVER

Fever is an elevated body temperature of more than 100.5°F, taken by mouth, that lasts for one or more days. Fever is usually caused by an infection. Infections can be viral (in which case the symptoms can be treated even though there may be no treatment for the cause), or they can be bacterial or fungal (in which case medicines may be prescribed after the infection is diagnosed). Other causes include inflammatory illness, drug reactions, or tumor growth. Sometimes, the cause may not be known. With an infection, the fever is a result of the body "heating up" to try to kill any invading germs. A fever is an important natural defense against germs.

People undergoing chemotherapy are more likely to have infections because they have lower numbers of the white blood cells needed to fight infection. It is good to have an easy-to-read, easy-to-use, oral thermometer so you can check your body temperature. A person with a fever will feel warm to the touch and may feel tired and alternate between being warm and cold, sometimes having shaking chills. Other symptoms that can occur with a fever are body aches, skin rashes, and headaches.

WHAT THE PATIENT CAN DO

▸ Check your temperature by mouth or under your arm every two to three hours.

▸ Keep a record of your temperature readings.

▸ Drink a lot of liquids (for example, water, fruit juices, cola, ice pops, and soups).

▸ Get enough rest.

▸ Keep layered bedding available to deal with temperature changes.

▸ Use a cold compress on your forehead if you are hot.

- Take acetaminophen (Tylenol) or other medicines for fever if prescribed by the doctor.

WHAT CAREGIVERS CAN DO

- Watch for shaking chills, and check the patient's temperature after the shaking stops.
- Check the patient's temperature by placing the thermometer in the mouth or under the arm. Do not take the temperature rectally unless the doctor tells you it's okay.
- Do not allow people who have fevers or any contagious illness to visit the patient. Encourage these potential visitors to call the patient until they are well again.
- Offer extra fluids and snacks.
- Help the patient take medicines on schedule.

CALL THE DOCTOR if the patient has any of these symptoms:

- A fever of 100.5 or higher, for temperature taken by mouth
- Fever lasting more than twenty-four hours
- Shaking chills
- Inability to drink fluids
- Confusion
- Disorientation
- Forgetfulness
- Two or more of the symptoms below, which can be signs of an infection—
  - New areas of redness or swelling
  - New cough or shortness of breath
  - New abdominal pain
  - Sore throat
  - Pain with urination
  - Pus or yellowish discharge from an injury or other location

Fluids and Dehydration

Everything in the body contains fluid (water). The human body must have a certain amount of liquid to function, so reduced amounts of fluid in the body can cause changes in the way a person feels. Fluid balance means that the body's fluids are properly regulated and in the proper places. Swelling is too much water in the body. Dehydration is not having enough water in the body or not having enough fluid where it is needed in the body.

These are the signs of dehydration:

▶ Dry mouth, thirst

▶ Dizziness, weakness

▶ Constipation

▶ Difficulty swallowing dry food

▶ Difficulty talking because of dry or sticky tissues in the mouth

▶ Dry skin, skin that "tents" (stays up) when pinched

▶ Swollen, cracked, or dry tongue

▶ Fever

▶ Weight loss

▶ Little or no urine

▶ Fatigue

▶ Sunken eyeballs

WHAT THE PATIENT CAN DO

▶ Drink fluids, such as water, juices, and colas. Sometimes iced fluids are easier to drink.

- Remember that food contains fluid. Try to eat fruits, vegetables, soups, gelatins, and other moist foods.
- Apply lotion often to ease dry skin, and apply a lubricant to lips to avoid painful cracking.
- Try to eliminate the cause of dehydration, such as vomiting, diarrhea, or fever. (See the related sections in this book for more information on these issues.)
- Use ice chips for relief of dry mouth if you can't drink enough liquid.

WHAT CAREGIVERS CAN DO

- Offer the patient cold or cool liquids every hour or so. If it is tiring for the patient to get up, fill a small cooler with ice and small cans of juice and keep it next to the bed or sofa.
- Encourage the patient to eat small meals if the patient is able to eat.
- Include moist foods, soups, and fruit smoothies (made with ice in a blender) as snacks.
- Check the patient's urine output to watch for dark color or to see if patient stops urinating.
- Watch for signs of confusion.
- Stand by when he or she gets up, in case of dizziness or fainting.

CALL THE DOCTOR if the patient has any of these symptoms:

- Vomiting, diarrhea, or fever that lasts for more than twenty-four hours
- Urine that is very dark in color, passing only a small amount of urine, or no urine for twelve hours or more
- Dizziness or faintness when standing up
- Confusion or disorientation

GROOMING AND APPEARANCE

Caring for your appearance can help you feel better about yourself. It is especially important when you are ill, because it can be harder to feel good about yourself when you are sick. In addition to routine hygiene, you may want to put extra time and energy into the way you look. Looking your best can help you feel more confident and in control.

WHAT THE PATIENT CAN DO

▸ Keep up with your regular grooming activities such as shaving, putting on makeup, and fixing your hair, even if you are confined to bed.

▸ If you will need a wig or toupee, see the section on hair loss on page 49 for suggestions on where to start.

▸ Have clothes altered if you lose or gain weight.

▸ Pamper yourself. Have a manicure or pedicure, facial, massage, or something else that makes you feel good. (Check with your doctor or nurse first.)

▸ Use an electric razor for routine shaving to prevent nicks and cuts.

▸ Exercise each day, but only as much as you can manage comfortably. Ask your doctor or nurse about an exercise plan, or just take slow, easy walks.

▸ Get enough rest.

▸ Keep up with regular dental care.

WHAT CAREGIVERS CAN DO

▸ When the patient is strong enough, encourage short outings that he or she can enjoy.

▸ Help the patient keep a supply of favorite toiletries, lotions, and grooming supplies on hand.

Hair Loss

The normal scalp contains about 100,000 hairs. They are constantly growing, with old hairs falling out and being replaced by new ones. Some cancer treatments will cause people to lose some or all of their hair, most often in clumps during shampooing or brushing. Sometimes clumps of hair are found on the pillow in the morning.

It is normal to feel distressed about hair loss. It helps to understand why it happens, to know that hair will grow back, and to take steps to make it less of a problem. Hair loss can happen when chemotherapy drugs travel throughout the body to kill cancer cells. Some of these drugs damage hair follicles, causing the hair to fall out. Hair loss can be hard to predict. Some patients have it and others do not, even when they take the same drugs. Some drugs can cause hair loss on the scalp and other places on the body, while some will cause only the loss of hair from the scalp. Radiation therapy to the head often causes scalp hair loss. Sometimes, depending on the dose of radiation to the head, the hair does not grow back the same as it was before treatment.

If hair loss does occur, it usually begins within two weeks of the start of treatment and gets worse one to two months after starting therapy. The scalp may feel very sensitive to washing, combing, or brushing during the short time when the hair is actually falling out. Hair often starts to grow back even before therapy is completed.

WHAT THE PATIENT CAN DO

▸ Be gentle when brushing and washing your hair. Hair loss can be reduced somewhat by avoiding too much brushing or pulling of hair and by avoiding heat (produced by electric rollers, hair dryers, and curling irons).

- Avoid styles that pull on the hair, such as braids or ponytails.

- Wear a hair net at night, or sleep on a satin pillowcase to minimize the effects of hair loss.

- Use a wide-toothed comb.

- Be gentle with your eyelashes and eyebrows, which may also be affected by treatment.

- If you are bothered by hair falling out, you may choose to shave your head.

- If you think you might want a wig, buy it before treatment begins or at the very start of treatment. (Ask if the wig can be adjusted—your wig size can shrink as you lose hair.) If you buy a wig before hair loss begins, the wig shop can better match your hair color and texture. Or you can cut a swatch of hair from the top front of your head, where hair is lightest, to use for matching.

- Be sure to get a prescription from your doctor for the wig—wigs are often covered by insurance.

- Get a list of wig shops in your area from your doctor or nurse, other patients, or from the phone book. You can also order a *tlc*™ catalog (a catalog of products for women undergoing cancer treatment) by calling 800-850-9445, or by visiting the Web site: www.tlcdirect.org.

- When selecting a wig, try on different styles until you find one that you really like. Consider buying two wigs, one for everyday and one for special occasions.

- Synthetic wigs need less styling than human hair wigs. They may be more manageable if you have low energy during cancer treatment.

- Turbans or scarves can be used instead of wigs. Cotton items tend to stay on your smooth scalp better than nylon or polyester.

- ▸ If you choose not to wear a wig, wear a hat or scarf outdoors in cold weather to reduce the loss of body heat. Use sunscreen, sunblock, or a hat to protect your scalp from the sun.

- ▸ When new hair starts to grow, it may easily break at first. Avoid perms for the first few months. Keep hair short and easy to style.

Health Insurance

Health insurance helps cover the cost of the diagnosis and treatment of cancer. In the past, most people in the United States had private, fee-for-service (indemnity) insurance. This meant that a person could go to any doctor or hospital, and the insurance company and the patient would each pay part of the bill. Today, more than half of Americans who have health insurance are enrolled in some type of managed care plan, another way of providing and paying for health care services.

For those who are sixty-five or older, coverage may be offered through Medicare, a federal insurance program. People with Medicare are now offered either managed care or indemnity plans. Medicaid, a joint federal-state health insurance program that is run by the states, covers some low-income people (especially women and children) and disabled people. Each state chooses the type of health plan to offer potential Medicaid patients. Veterans may receive benefits through a Veterans Administration (VA) program.

Whatever the type of insurance you have, you will want to get the most from your plan. You will get the best care if you stay informed and know about the benefits, coverage, and limits of your plan. Take charge of your care by asking questions. Be involved in making decisions about your care, and keep track of the care you receive.

WHAT THE PATIENT CAN DO

▸ Do not let your health insurance expire.

▸ Get a copy of your health insurance policy and find out what it covers, especially as it relates to your cancer and treatment.

- If you have a job with health insurance benefits, keep it until you have a new job with the coverage you need.

- If you are unable to work for a time, talk with your employer about ways to keep your health insurance. For instance, the Family and Medical Leave Act (FMLA), paid or unpaid time off, or temporary disability benefits may be helpful.

- If your health insurance requires claims, send in claims for all covered costs. Keep careful records of all your health care expenses and all claims submitted, pending, and paid. Follow up with your insurance company if you have questions about filed claims. If a claim is denied, submit it again.

- Find out if a case manager has been assigned to you by your insurance company. Get to know this person and keep him or her informed of what is happening with your treatment. This person can help you through many of the health insurance issues that may come up.

- Work with your doctor's office staff or the hospital billing department to get the most coverage you can. If your cancer care team has a social worker, talk with him or her about your insurance and job situation.

- Consider filing an insurance complaint if you feel you have been treated unfairly.

- Look for other options for getting insurance after cancer treatment. Consider joining your state's "high risk" health insurance pool for people who cannot get regular health coverage, using Medicare or Medicaid, getting dependent coverage under your spouse's insurance plan, joining your current company plan, getting coverage through an independent broker, or getting group insurance through an organization you've joined.

- Keep your insurance needs in mind if you think about getting a new job.

▸ Help the patient track insurance claims for treatments, drugs, and hospitals. You may need to handle the paperwork during times that the patient is very weak or sick.

▸ Keep the phone numbers of the patient's employer's benefits department, insurance companies, and claim agents in a handy place. Or keep all the insurance information in one notebook or binder.

HICCUPS

Hiccups happen when the diaphragm (the main muscle used in breathing) suddenly contracts between normal breaths. Hiccups can be caused by irritation of the nerve that controls the diaphragm, certain drugs, problems in the brain, problems in the esophagus (the swallowing tube that goes from the throat to the stomach), pressure on the stomach, and other conditions.

Hiccups that last a long time can be serious. They can interfere with eating, sleeping, and breathing and can lead to exhaustion.

WHAT THE PATIENT CAN DO

▶ Breathe slowly and deeply into a paper bag for ten breaths at a time.

▶ Drink water slowly.

▶ Hold a teaspoon of sugar in your mouth and then swallow.

▶ Avoid forcing yourself to eat, as this might cause vomiting.

WHAT CAREGIVERS CAN DO

▶ Watch the patient to be sure that he or she is able to drink enough liquids.

▶ If medicine is given for hiccups, watch for dizziness. The patient may need help getting up or walking.

 CALL THE DOCTOR if the patient has trouble breathing, develops a puffy or bloated stomach, or has hiccups that last for more than one day.

Hospice Care

Hospice programs provide supportive care for the patient and the family in the final stages of disease—that is, the last days, weeks, or months of life. Hospice care can be provided in the home, in hospitals that have hospice units, or in free-standing hospice facilities. Hospice care seeks to make the patient as comfortable as possible, relieve symptoms, and help the patient and family have the best possible quality of life.

Some people prefer to die at home, while others feel better in a hospital setting. There are no right or wrong choices, only personal ones that are best for you and your family. Hospice works with the family to provide care and to meet the physical, functional, emotional, and spiritual needs of the patient. Accepting death is central to the hospice approach, although the focus is on caring for and supporting the patient, helping him or her to live as fully as possible until death.

Whatever the setting, hospice care is offered widely. It is covered by Medicare, Medicaid, and most insurance plans.

WHAT THE PATIENT CAN DO

- Find out if your insurance plan covers hospice care.
- Sort through your feelings and your family's feelings about dying at home.
- Ask to speak to someone from local hospice programs and have them discuss the type of care they can offer.

WHAT CAREGIVERS CAN DO

- If home hospice is planned, find out how they would care for the patient and what would be expected of you and your family. Talk honestly with the hospice staff about any concerns you have.

▸ Remember that illnesses unrelated to cancer can still be treated if it will make the patient more comfortable.

▸ After the patient has been enrolled in hospice care, keep the phone numbers for the nurse, social worker, chaplain, and others handy. Keep the nurse informed about any changes in the patient's physical condition, unrelieved pain, or any problems the patient has.

When Death Is Approaching

You may be with your loved one at the time of death. The following section looks at the process of dying and describes some signs that death may be close. Not all of the following symptoms will happen, but it may be comforting to know about them. People often use this time to gather the family to say goodbye to their loved one. They may take turns with the patient, holding hands, talking to the patient, or just sitting quietly. It can also be a time to perform any religious rituals or other activities the patient wants before death. It is a chance for many families and friends to express their love and appreciation for the patient and for each other.

It is important to have a plan for what to do after death, so that the family knows what to do during this very emotional time. The hospice nurse and social worker will know what steps need to be taken and can help you.

These are some of the signs the patient is nearing death:

▸ Profound weakness—usually the patient cannot get out of bed and has trouble moving around in bed.

▸ The patient needs help with nearly everything he or she does.

▸ There is less and less interest in food, often with very little food and fluid intake for days.

- Drowsiness will increase—the patient may doze or sleep much of the time if pain is relieved. He or she may be hard to rouse or wake.

- The patient may be restless and pick or pull at bed linens. Anxiety, fear, restlessness, and loneliness may worsen at night.

- The patient cannot concentrate or has a short attention span. He or she is confused about time, place, or people.

- Swallowing pills and medicines is difficult.

- He or she has a limited ability to cooperate with caregivers.

Possible Changes in Body Function

- The patient will be weak.

- He or she has trouble moving around in bed and may not be able to get out of bed.

- The patient cannot change positions without help.

- Swallowing food, medicines, or even liquids will be difficult.

- There may be sudden movement of muscles, jerking of hands, arms, legs, or face.

WHAT CAREGIVERS CAN DO

- Help the patient turn and change positions every hour or two.

- Avoid sudden noises or movements to lessen the patient's startle reflex.

- Speak in a calm, quiet voice to reduce the chances of startling the patient.

- If the patient has trouble swallowing pain medicines, ask the doctor or hospice nurse about liquid pain medicines or the pain patch.

- If the patient is having trouble swallowing, avoid giving him or her solid foods. Give ice chips or sips of liquid through a straw.

- Do not push fluids. Near the end of life, some dehydration is normal and is more comfortable for the patient.

- Apply cool, moist washcloths to the head, face, and body for comfort.

Possible Changes in Consciousness

- The patient sleeps more during the day and is hard to wake or rouse from sleep.

- The patient is confused about time, place, or people. He or she may talk about things unrelated to the events or people present.

- He or she is restless and may pick or pull at bed linens. Restlessness, anxiety, fear, and loneliness may be worse at night.

- After a period of sleepiness and confusion, the patient may have a short time when he or she is mentally clear before going back into a semiconscious state.

WHAT CAREGIVERS CAN DO

- Plan your time with the patient for when he or she is most alert or during the night when your presence may be comforting.

- When talking with the patient, remind him or her who you are and what day and time it is.

- Continue the patient's pain medicines up to the end of life.

- If the patient is very restless, try to find out if he or she is having pain. If it appears so, give "breakthrough" pain medicines as prescribed, or check with the doctor or hospice nurse, if needed. (See the section on pain on page 82.)

- When talking with a confused person, use calm, confident, gentle tones to reduce the chances of startling or frightening the patient.

- ▸ Touching, caressing, holding, and rocking the patient are usually helpful and comforting.

Possible Changes in Metabolism

- ▸ The patient has less interest in and need for food and drink.

- ▸ His or her mouth may dry out. (See the section on possible changes in secretions below.)

- ▸ The patient may no longer need some of his or her medicines, such as vitamins, chemotherapy, replacement hormones, blood pressure medicines, and diuretics, unless they help make the patient more comfortable.

WHAT CAREGIVERS CAN DO

- ▸ Apply lubricant or petroleum jelly (Vaseline) to the patient's lips to prevent drying.

- ▸ Ice chips from a spoon or sips of water or juice from a straw may be enough for the patient.

- ▸ Check with the doctor to see which medicines may be stopped. Medicines for pain, nausea, fever, seizures, or anxiety should be continued to keep the patient comfortable.

Possible Changes in Secretions

- ▸ Mucus in the mouth may collect in the back of the throat. This can be a very distressing sound to hear, but doesn't usually cause discomfort to the patient.

- ▸ Secretions may thicken because of lower fluid intake and build up because the patient cannot cough.

WHAT CAREGIVERS CAN DO

- ▸ If the patient's mouth secretions increase, keep them loose by adding humidity to the room with a cool mist humidifier.

- If the patient can swallow, ice chips or sips of liquid through a straw may thin the secretions.
- Change the patient's position—turning the patient to the side may help the secretions drain from the mouth. Continue to clean the patient's teeth with a soft toothbrush or soft foam mouth swabs.
- Certain medicines may help the patient—ask your hospice or home care nurse.

Possible Changes in Circulation and Temperature

- The arms and legs may feel cool to the touch as circulation slows down.
- The skin of the patient's arms, legs, hands, and feet may darken in color and appear mottled.
- Other areas of the body may become either darker or more pale.
- The patient's skin may feel cold and either dry or damp.
- The patient's heart rate may become fast, faint, or irregular.
- The patient's blood pressure may get lower and become hard to hear.

WHAT CAREGIVERS CAN DO

- Keep the patient warm with blankets or light bed coverings.
- Avoid using electric blankets, heating pads, etc.

Possible Changes in Senses and Perception

- The patient's vision may become blurry or dim.
- Hearing may decrease, but most patients are able to hear you even after they can no longer speak.

▶ Leave on indirect lights as vision decreases.

▶ Never assume the patient cannot hear you.

▶ Continue to speak with and touch the patient to reassure him or her of your presence. Your words of affection and support are likely to be understood and appreciated.

Possible Changes in Breathing

▶ Breathing may speed up and slow down because of lower blood circulation and buildup of waste products in the body.

▶ Mucus in the back of the patient's throat may cause rattling or gurgling with each breath.

▶ The patient may not breathe for periods of ten to thirty seconds.

WHAT CAREGIVERS CAN DO

▶ Put the patient on his or her back or slightly to one side.

▶ Raising the patient's head may provide some relief.

▶ Use pillows to prop the patient's head and chest at an angle or raise the head of a hospital bed.

▶ Any position that seems to make breathing easier is okay, including sitting up with good support. A small person may be more comfortable in your arms.

Possible Changes in Elimination

▶ Amounts of urine may decrease and may be darker in color.

▶ When death is near, the patient may lose control of urine and stool.

WHAT CAREGIVERS CAN DO

▸ Pad the bed beneath the patient with layers of disposable waterproof pads.

▸ If the patient has a catheter, the home health care nurse will teach you to take care of it.

When death does occur, breathing stops and the patient's blood pressure cannot be heard. The pulse will stop, and the eyes will stop moving and may stay open. The pupils of the eyes will stay large, even in bright light. Control of the bowels and bladder is lost as the muscles relax.

After death, it is okay to sit with your loved one for a while. There is no rush to get anything done right away. Many families find this is an important time to pray or talk together and reconfirm your love for each other, as well as for the person who has passed away.

If the patient dies in the home, caregivers are responsible for calling the proper people. Regulations or laws about who must be notified and how the body should be removed differ from one community to another. Your doctor or nurse can get this information for you. If you have a hospice or home care agency involved, call them. If you have completed funeral arrangements, the only remaining tasks will be to call the funeral director and doctor.

For more information on what to expect when death is approaching, contact the American Cancer Society at 800-ACS-2345 and ask for *Nearing the End of Life*. More information is also available on the Web at www.cancer.org. More information on hospice care is available from the American Cancer Society or the National Hospice and Palliative Care Organization (NHPCO) at 800-658-8898 (Hospice Helpline) or www.nhpco.org.

IMMUNOTHERAPY

Immunotherapy is a promising type of treatment for certain cancers. It is sometimes called biologic therapy, biotherapy, or biological response modifier therapy. These therapies use different parts of the body's immune system to fight cancer or lessen the side effects of some cancer treatments.

Immunotherapies can act in several ways in cancer treatment. For instance, they may slow or stop the growth of cancer cells. They may help healthy cells, especially immune system cells that control cancer. They may also help repair or replace normal cells damaged by other cancer treatments.

There are different kinds of immunotherapy now in use. You may hear terms such as interferons, interleukins, cytokines, monoclonal antibodies, or tumor necrosis factor. If you are having immunotherapy, ask your doctor to explain what kind it is and how the medicine works. More than one kind of immunotherapy may be used at different times or together. It may also be used along with chemotherapy or radiation treatment. Some types of immunotherapy have been in use for years, while others are fairly new.

If you are not receiving immunotherapy, you may want to ask your doctor or cancer care team if it is an option for your type of cancer. Many of these treatments are being studied today to learn how well they work and how safe they are. Your doctor or cancer care team will be able to tell you more about clinical trials using immunotherapy.

WHAT THE PATIENT CAN DO

▶ Ask questions. Your cancer care team will help you.

▶ Consider getting a second opinion before starting a new immunotherapy.

- Ask about expected side effects and how to cope with them.
- Find out when you should call your doctor.
- Go to every scheduled appointment.
- If you are having other symptoms, such as fatigue, see the related sections in this book and inform your doctor or nurse.

WHAT CAREGIVERS CAN DO

- Find out how to reach the doctor when his or her office is closed.
- Watch for confusion or dizziness.
- Keep a list of questions to ask the doctor or care team. It may help to make notes of problems that the patient may forget.
- If the patient is fatigued, nauseated, or vomiting, refer to the related sections in this book on how to deal with these effects.

 CALL THE DOCTOR if the patient develops a fever, has severe nausea and vomiting, gets dizzy or has trouble breathing, or becomes confused or disoriented.

ITCHING

Itching can cause restlessness, anxiety, skin sores, and infection. Common causes in people with cancer include dry skin, changes in the blood, allergies, the side effects of medicines, and chemotherapy or radiation therapy. Other illnesses and certain kinds of cancer can also cause itching. The skin can become dry, red, rough, and flaky, and the patient may develop a rash or bumps on the skin. Sometimes the patient will scratch without realizing it; excessive scratching can lead to skin sores and scratch marks.

WHAT THE PATIENT CAN DO

▸ Apply skin creams with a water-soluble base, such as aloe vera or menthol-based lotion, two to three times a day—especially after bathing when the skin is damp. Calamine lotion or witch hazel may soothe the itching, but note that they can cause dryness.

▸ Use warm instead of hot water for bathing.

▸ Add baking soda, oatmeal (in a cloth or mesh bag), or bath oil to your bath water.

▸ Wash your skin gently using a mild, unscented soap.

▸ Use baking soda instead of deodorant.

▸ Avoid using scented or alcohol-based products (such as powder, aftershave lotion, or perfume) on the skin. Cornstarch-based powders may clump in moist areas and cause irritation.

▸ Use an electric razor for shaving rather than a blade to avoid irritation.

▸ Drink as much water and other fluids as you can.

▸ Get enough rest.

- To reduce the desire to scratch, apply a cool pack (crushed ice in a plastic bag wrapped in a towel) to the skin. Remove it when it becomes warm and let your skin warm. Use as needed.
- Keep nails clean and short. Wear clean cotton gloves if you scratch without thinking about it.
- Try relieving the itching with rubbing, pressure, cool cloths, or vibration instead of scratching. Avoid breaking the skin. Get massages at night.
- Wear loose clothing made of soft fabric.
- Distract yourself with music, reading, and the company of others.
- Take medicines for itching as prescribed by your doctor.

WHAT CAREGIVERS CAN DO

- Try using mild, unscented detergents to wash clothes and bedding.
- If the patient scratches in his or her sleep, clean cotton gloves may reduce skin damage.
- Offer to give the patient massages—they may help to relieve the itching.
- Try to distract the patient by spending time together doing activities he or she enjoys.
- Keep the patient's room cool (60° to 70°F) and well ventilated.
- Change the patient's bed sheets daily.

CALL THE DOCTOR if the patient has any of these symptoms:

- Itching that does not go away after two or more days

- A yellowish color to the skin or eyes or tea-colored urine

- Open wounds due to scratching

- A rash that gets worse after creams or ointments have been applied

- A foul-smelling drainage or pus from the skin

- Anxiety and restlessness due to itching, to the point that the patient cannot sleep through the night

- Hives (itchy white or red welts on the skin), shortness of breath, swelling of the throat or face, or other symptoms of severe allergic reaction

Leg Cramps

Leg cramps or spasms are a painful tightening of the muscles in the leg. Staying in bed for long periods can sometimes cause muscles in the leg or foot to cramp. Dehydration, certain drugs, and brain or nerve diseases can also cause this reaction. Other causes of cramping include pressure on the calf muscles or the back of the knee or chemical imbalances in the blood, such as too much phosphorus, too little calcium, low blood sugar, or too little potassium. The cramp will cause sudden pain or discomfort and a tight or stiff feeling in the leg or foot. The patient may have trouble moving the foot or pain when moving the foot or leg.

WHAT THE PATIENT CAN DO

▸ If you are bed-bound, change your position often.

▸ Use a bed cradle to protect the legs and feet from the weight of the bedclothes. A bed cradle is a support at the end of the bed that holds up the sheets and blanket to avoid touching the legs and feet.

▸ Keep warm.

▸ Exercise your legs in bed by bending and straightening them ten times twice a day or as many times as you can. A caregiver can move your legs for you if you cannot.

▸ Tell your doctor or nurse about the cramps. There are ways to prevent cramps. The doctor may prescribe a muscle relaxer.

▸ Apply heat to legs in spasm, if allowed by your doctor. Talk to your doctor or nurse about what kind of heat to use and how long you should use it.

▸ You can also try using ice and gently rub the cramped muscle.

- Massage the tight muscle, if allowed by your doctor.
- Contract the opposite muscle group to stretch the tight muscle as much as you can without hurting it. For example, for a calf muscle cramp, try pointing the toes upward toward the knees or walking around.
- Follow your doctor's instructions for correcting imbalances in calcium, potassium, or phosphorus.

WHAT CAREGIVERS CAN DO

- Help the patient exercise the legs if he or she has trouble moving them. Bend and straighten the legs ten times twice a day.
- Help the patient stretch the tight muscle if he or she cannot.
- If muscle relaxers are used, watch for dizziness or stumbling.

CALL THE DOCTOR if the patient has any of these symptoms:

- Cramping that is not relieved by heat, ice, massage, or stretching the cramped muscle
- Cramping that lasts for more than six to eight hours
- A cramped leg that becomes red, swollen, or hot

Mouth Bleeding

Bleeding in the mouth is generally caused by mouth sores, gum (periodontal) disease, or by a low number of platelets (cells that help the blood to clot). Low platelet counts can be a side effect of chemotherapy or radiation treatment. This is usually a temporary problem. Cancers that affect the blood-forming system, such as leukemia, can also cause a drop in platelets. A person with a low platelet count may bleed easily, and everyday actions such as brushing or flossing teeth can cause bleeding. Side effects of chemotherapy or radiation can include dryness in the mouth or small mouth ulcers, which can bleed. Watch for blood or bruises in the mouth, or a rash or red pinpoint-sized dots on the tongue, roof of the mouth, or inside of the cheeks.

WHAT THE PATIENT CAN DO

▸ Rinse your mouth gently with ice water every two hours.

▸ Have ice chips on hand to suck on. (Avoid hard candies if your mouth is bleeding.)

▸ Rinse your mouth or brush teeth with a soft toothbrush after eating. Soak the toothbrush in hot water before brushing to soften the bristles even more.

▸ If a soft toothbrush causes bleeding, use soft foam mouth swabs or gauze wrapped around a popsicle stick or tongue depressor to brush your teeth.

▸ Avoid store-bought mouthwash. See page 76 for how to make a gentle mouth rinse.

▸ Eat foods that are soft and smooth in consistency and high in calories and protein. (Refrigerated soft foods such as ice cream, applesauce, puddings, and yogurt are helpful because the cold helps control bleeding.)

- Put hard foods (such as apples, pears, etc.) in the blender.
- Avoid hot drinks such as coffee and tea. Heat enlarges blood vessels and can worsen bleeding.
- Apply cream or salve to lips to prevent dryness.
- If you normally wear dentures, do not wear them while you are having problems with mouth bleeding, especially if the dentures do not fit well.
- Avoid aspirin products. Check labels of over-the-counter drugs to be sure they don't contain aspirin, or check with your pharmacist.

WHAT CAREGIVERS CAN DO

- Offer cold water mouth rinses before each meal. Keep ice water nearby.
- If the patient's mouth is oozing blood, keep a bowl nearby for spitting out mouth rinses.
- Make milk shakes or smoothies in the blender, and offer other soft frozen treats. Avoid nuts, caramel, and hard coatings.
- Freeze a few wet tea bags, and have the patient press one on any area of bleeding.

CALL THE DOCTOR if the patient has any of these symptoms:

- Bleeding from the mouth for the first time
- Bleeding that lasts for more than thirty minutes
- Vomiting blood or material that looks like coffee grounds
- Feeling light-headed or dizzy

Mouth Dryness

Dry mouth occurs when there is not enough saliva in the mouth. It can be caused by breathing through the mouth or it may be a side effect of medicine, radiation treatment to the head and neck, or dehydration. The saliva may become thick like mucus, or there may be dried, flaky saliva in and around the mouth. The patient may have trouble swallowing food or thick liquids, and the tongue surface may appear ridged or cracked. Mouth dryness can also cause a burning sensation in the tongue and cause food particles to stick to the teeth, tongue, and gums.

WHAT THE PATIENT CAN DO

▸ Rinse your mouth every two hours with a salt and baking soda solution (one teaspoon of salt and one teaspoon of baking soda mixed with one quart of warm water). Shake before each use. Swish and spit. Do not swallow.

▸ Drink liquids with meals to moisten foods and to help with swallowing.

▸ Try ice chips, sugarless hard candies, and sugarless chewing gum.

▸ Add liquids to solid foods (e.g., gravy, sauce, milk, and yogurt).

▸ Use petroleum jelly, cocoa butter, or mild lip balm to keep your lips moist.

▸ Use artificial saliva, which is sold at drugstores.

▸ Avoid hot, spicy, or acidic foods; chewy candies; tough meats; and hard, raw fruits or vegetables.

▸ Avoid alcohol, including store-bought mouthwashes that contain alcohol.

▸ Avoid tobacco.

WHAT CAREGIVERS CAN DO

▶ Offer the patient small, soft meals with extra sauces.

▶ Offer the patient ice cream, gelatin, ice chips, and frozen drinks.

▶ Help the patient keep track of his or her fluid intake and encourage him or her to consume two or three quarts of liquid each day, if the doctor approves. Ice, ice cream, sherbet, ice pops, and gelatin count as liquids.

CALL THE DOCTOR if the patient has any of these symptoms:

- Dry mouth that lasts for more than three days
- Inability to take medicines or swallow pills
- Inability to drink or eat
- Dry, cracked lips or mouth sores
- Trouble breathing

MOUTH SORES

Mouth sores are like little cuts or ulcers in the mouth that can bleed or become infected. The sores may be very red or may have small white patches in the middle. They can appear one to two weeks after some kinds of chemotherapy. Mouth sores can also result from radiation treatments to the head and neck area, infection, dehydration, poor mouth care, oxygen therapy, alcohol or tobacco, not enough vitamins, or lack of protein. They can take two to four weeks to heal. Mouth sores can be very painful and can lead to dehydration, poor eating, and weight loss. The patient may have soft whitish patches or pus in the mouth, and the sores can cause feelings of dryness, mild burning, or pain when eating hot and cold foods. The patient may also have a white or yellow film in the mouth or on the tongue and increased mucus in the mouth. The inside of the mouth and gums will appear red, shiny, and swollen.

WHAT THE PATIENT CAN DO

▸ Check your mouth twice a day by using a small flashlight and a padded popsicle stick. If you wear dentures, take them out before you inspect your mouth. Report any changes in appearance, taste, or feeling to your doctor or nurse.

▸ Unless your doctor or nurse gives you other instructions, use the following plan for mouth care thirty minutes after eating and every four hours while you are awake (or at least twice a day):

- Brush your teeth using a soft, nylon-bristle toothbrush. To soften the bristles even more, soak the brush in hot water before brushing and rinse the brush with hot water during brushing. If the toothbrush hurts your mouth, use a popsicle stick with gauze wrapped around it or a cotton swab instead. You also can get soft foam mouth swabs from the drugstore.

- Rinse your toothbrush well in hot water after use and store in a cool, dry place.

- Use a nonabrasive toothpaste that contains fluoride. Note that whitening toothpastes may contain hydrogen peroxide, which can irritate mouth sores.

▶ If you wear dentures, remove and clean them regularly between meals. If you have sores under your dentures, leave your dentures out between meals and at night. Clean your dentures well between uses, and store them in an antibacterial soak. If your dentures fit poorly, do not use them during treatment.

▶ Gently rinse your mouth before and after meals and at bedtime with one of the following solutions: one teaspoon baking soda mixed with two cups water, or one teaspoon salt and one teaspoon baking soda dissolved in one quart of water.

▶ If you normally floss, continue to floss at least once a day unless you are told not to. Tell your doctor if this causes bleeding or other problems. If you did not floss regularly before treatment, talk with your doctor before you start.

▶ Avoid store-bought mouthwashes, which often contain alcohol or other irritants.

▶ Keep your lips moist with petroleum jelly, mild lip balm, or cocoa butter.

▶ Drink at least two to three quarts of fluids each day, if your doctor approves.

▶ If your mouth pain is severe or makes it hard to eat, ask your doctor about medicine that can be swished in the mouth fifteen to twenty minutes before meals or painted on each painful sore with a cotton swab before meals. If this does not work, you may need stronger pain medicine.

- Ask your doctor about using Maalox or Milk of Magnesia to help the sores heal. Allow the medicine to settle and separate, pour the liquid off the top of the solution, and swab the pasty part onto the sore area with a cotton swab. Rinse with water after fifteen to twenty minutes.
- Sip warm tea slowly.
- Eat chilled foods and fluids (ice pops, ice cubes, frozen yogurt, sherbet, ice cream, etc.).
- Eat small, frequent meals of bland, soft, moist foods that are easy to swallow. Avoid raw vegetables and fruits and other hard, dry, or crusty foods such as chips or pretzels.
- Avoid very salty or high-sugar foods.
- Avoid acidic fruits and juices, such as tomato, orange, grapefruit, lime, or lemon.
- Avoid fizzy drinks, alcohol, and tobacco.

WHAT CAREGIVERS CAN DO

- Use a flashlight to check the patient's mouth for red areas or white patches, which often become sores. If the patient wears dentures, remove them first.
- Offer the patient liquids with a straw, which may help bypass the sore areas in the mouth.
- Mash or purée hard foods in a blender to make them easier to eat.
- Try coating mouth sores with Anbesol before meals to numb them during eating.
- Offer the patient pain medicines half an hour before mealtime.
- Try to create a pleasant mealtime atmosphere.

CALL THE DOCTOR if the patient has any of these symptoms:

- Redness or shininess in mouth that lasts for more than forty-eight hours
- Bleeding gums
- Any type of cut or sore in the mouth
- Fever of 100.5°F or higher, for temperature taken by mouth
- White patches on the tongue or inside the mouth
- Little intake of food or fluid for two days
- Inability to take medicines because of mouth sores

Nausea and Vomiting

Nausea is having a sick or queasy feeling in the stomach, and vomiting is throwing up food or liquids from the stomach. Nausea can occur even when a person is not thinking about food. A person can vomit even if he or she has not eaten anything and hasn't had any nausea. Nausea and vomiting can be caused by eating something that disagrees with you, bacteria in food, infections, or by radiation or chemotherapy treatments for cancer. Many people have little or no nausea and vomiting with these treatments. For others, just thinking about having one of the treatments can cause nausea or vomiting. Cancer by itself may also cause nausea and vomiting. Patients may experience increased saliva, clamminess, and sweating before vomiting. Frequent vomiting can be dangerous because it can lead to dehydration. It can also cause choking or inhaling of food or liquids. Talk with your doctor about what is causing your nausea and vomiting and what you can do about it.

WHAT THE PATIENT CAN DO

For nausea:

▸ Eat bland foods, such as dry toast and crackers.

▸ If the nausea only happens between meals, eat frequent, small meals and have a snack at bedtime.

▸ Drink clear liquids like ginger ale, apple juice, or broth, served cold and sipped slowly. You can also try frozen ice pops or gelatin.

▸ Seek out the foods you like. Many people develop a dislike for red meat and meat broths. Try other protein sources such as fish, chicken, beans, and nuts.

▸ Eat food cold or at room temperature to decrease its smell and taste. Avoid fatty, fried, spicy, or very sweet foods.

- Try eating small amounts of foods that are high in calories and easy to eat (pudding, ice cream, sherbets, yogurt, milk shakes, etc.) several times a day. Use butter, oils, syrups, and milk in foods to raise calories. Avoid low-fat foods unless fats upset your stomach or cause other problems.

- Tart or sour foods may be easier to keep down (unless you have mouth sores).

- Suck on hard candy with a pleasant smell, such as lemon drops or mints, to help get rid of bad tastes.

- Try to rest quietly while sitting upright for at least an hour after each meal.

- Distract yourself with soft music, a favorite television program, or the company of others.

- If you have nausea, relax and take slow deep breaths.

- Be sure your doctor is aware of your nausea—there are several drugs that can help it.

- As directed by your doctor, take any anti-nausea medicine at the first hint of nausea to prevent vomiting.

- If nausea occurs just before doctor visits, ask about medicines, hypnosis, relaxation, exercises or behavioral treatments to lessen this problem.

For vomiting:

- If you are in bed, lie on your side so that vomit will not be inhaled.

- Request that medicines be prescribed in suppository form, if possible. Take any anti-nausea medicine at the first hint of nausea to prevent vomiting.

- Try liquids in the form of ice chips or frozen juice chips that can be taken slowly.

- After vomiting stops, begin by taking in one teaspoon of cool liquid every ten minutes. Gradually increase to one tablespoon every half hour. If you are able to keep that down after an hour or so, try larger amounts.

WHAT CAREGIVERS CAN DO

▸ Make meals or ask others to make meals during times the patient is nauseated. Use the kitchen vent fan to reduce odors. Cover or remove foods with strong or unpleasant odors.

▸ Have the patient try plastic forks and spoons rather than metal ones, which may cause a bitter taste.

▸ If the patient is vomiting, weigh him or her at the same time each day, to help determine whether dehydration is getting severe.

▸ Talk to the doctor about medicines to help prevent vomiting.

▸ Watch the patient for dizziness, weakness, or confusion.

▸ Try to help the patient avoid constipation and dehydration. Either of these can make nausea worse. See pages 26 and 46 for more about these problems.

CALL THE DOCTOR if the patient has any of these symptoms:

- Has inhaled any of the vomited material

- Vomiting more than three times an hour for three or more hours

- Vomiting blood or material that looks like coffee grounds

- Inability to take in more than four cups of liquid or ice chips in a day or eat substantial foods for more than two days

- Inability to take his or her medicines

- Weakness, dizziness, or confusion

- Loss of two or more pounds in one to two days, which can mean he or she is losing too much water

- Dark yellow urine or a decrease in urination

Pain

When people say they are having pain, it usually means they are hurting somewhere in their body. But it can also mean that they just can't get comfortable. They may be feeling bad in general, not in any one specific place. Pain can be worse if a person is anxious, sad, or depressed. Some people may have a hard time talking about pain. Their reluctance can be due to the way they were brought up, the way people in their family express themselves, or an aspect of their individual personality. In general, the way the patient talked about pain in the past, before the illness, will be the way they talk about it now.

Even severe pain can be very well controlled by combinations of medicines that can be taken by mouth. These combinations usually include opioids (OH-pee-oyds) such as morphine or codeine. The body can become tolerant of the pain medicine after a time, so the dose may need to be increased to get the same pain relief. This is a common sign of opioid tolerance.

Note that addiction is not usually a concern in people with cancer who take opioid pain-relieving drugs. Nor is it a sign of addiction when a cancer patient who takes opioids needs increased doses to get relief.

Pain medicines work best if they are used around the clock, before the pain becomes severe. It takes more medicine to control severe pain than milder pain, so it's best to treat pain as soon as it starts and regularly after that. If the cause of the pain is treated, the need for medicine will slowly decrease or disappear. Drug dosages and schedules should be adjusted by the doctor as the patient's needs change.

Pain from cancer that has spread or other long-term cancer pain can exhaust you. This type of chronic or long-term pain can interfere with your life and keep you from doing the things you want and need to do. Even with around-the-clock pain medicines, pain often "breaks through" between doses. Breakthrough pain usually calls for a second pain medicine that you can take safely in addition to your regular pain medicine. Don't be surprised if it takes more than two medicines to control your pain. Help your doctor keep your pain under control by taking pain medicines as prescribed and keeping him informed about your level of pain.

Watch for whether the pain ever goes away. If it goes away for a while, but comes back before the next dose is due, the medicine plan may need to be changed. Pain can cause the patient to have trouble sleeping or cause a lack of interest in things he or she used to enjoy. Pain can also hamper the patient's ability to move around. It may cause worry about things that did not cause concern in the past.

WHAT THE PATIENT CAN DO

▸ Talk with your doctor or nurse about your pain—where the pain is, when it began, how long it lasts, what it feels like, what makes it better, what makes it worse, and how it affects your life.

▸ If the prescribed pain medicines don't work as expected, let your doctor or nurse know.

▸ Rate your pain using a pain rating scale, for example, where zero equals no pain and ten equals the worst pain you can imagine. You can use this scale to explain your pain to others.

▸ Take your pain medicine exactly as prescribed. Do not wait until the pain is severe before taking pain medicine. For chronic pain, medicine should be given around the clock on a schedule rather than only when pain is severe. Check with your doctor if this schedule needs to be adjusted.

▸ As the pain is relieved with medicines, increase your activity level.

- Avoid suddenly stopping any of your pain medicines. Talk with your doctor, nurse, or pharmacist before you reduce the dosage or if you have questions.

- Some people feel nauseated even when taking the right dose of pain medicine. Ask your doctor to change the pain medicine or give you something to control the nausea.

- Some pain medicines make you drowsy or dizzy. This often lessens after a few days, but you may need help getting up or walking. Don't try to drive or do anything dangerous until you are sure of the effects.

- People receiving opioid pain medicines are normally given laxatives and stool softeners to prevent constipation, which is a common side effect of opioids.

- Keep track of any other side effects you notice. Discuss them with your doctor or nurse.

- Avoid crushing or breaking your pain pills unless you check with your doctor, nurse, or pharmacist. If your medicines are in time-release form, taking broken pills can be dangerous.

- If pain medicines are not keeping your pain under control, talk with the doctor about other measures. If you continue to have trouble, ask to see a pain specialist.

- Keep at least one week's supply of pain medicines on hand. Most pain medicines cannot be refilled by telephone, so you will need a written prescription.

WHAT CAREGIVERS CAN DO

- Watch the patient for signs of unrelieved pain. Ask about pain if you notice grimacing, moaning, tension, or reluctance to move around in bed.

- Try warm baths or warm washcloths on painful areas, avoiding areas where radiation was given. If this doesn't help, you can try ice or cool packs. Massage or applying pressure may help some types of pain.

- Talk with the doctor or nurse so that you understand what medicines are for pain and how each is to be used.

- If the patient is having trouble taking pills, talk with the doctor about medicines that come in different forms, such as liquids, suppositories, or skin patches.

- Check with the doctor, nurse, or pharmacist before you crush or dissolve pain pills to make them easier to swallow. Some pills can cause a dangerous overdose if broken.

- Remind the patient that pain medicine, when used as directed, does not cause addiction.

- Be sure you have a list of all the medicines the patient is taking, including pain medicines. This is even more important if unexpected medical problems come up.

- Keep opioid pain medicines away from others, especially children and pets.

- Watch for confusion and dizziness, especially after new medicines are started or when doses are changed. Help the patient with walking until you know he or she can do it safely.

- Encourage pleasant distractions that the patient enjoys.

- Plan activities for when the patient is most comfortable and awake.

- Offer the patient plenty of fluids and food with fiber. Help the patient remember to take stool softeners and laxatives the doctor suggests to prevent constipation. See page 26 for more about preventing constipation.

- If the patient seems forgetful, help him or her track when pain medicines are due to avoid over- or under-dosing.

- If the patient is having frequent, severe pain, talk with the doctor about medicine to take around the clock. If pain "breaks through," find out if there is another medicine to use between doses of the main pain medicine.

- Know how to reach the doctor when his or her office is closed.

- Plan time for activities you enjoy, and take care of yourself. A support group for family members may be helpful.

CALL THE DOCTOR if the patient has any of these symptoms:

- New or more severe pain
- Inability to take anything by mouth, including pain medicine
- No pain relief or relief that doesn't last long enough with prescribed medicines
- Difficulty waking up or staying awake
- Constipation, nausea, or confusion
- Any new symptom (for example, an inability to walk, eat, or urinate)

For more in-depth information on pain management, call the American Cancer Society at 800-ACS-2345 and ask for a copy of *Pain Control: A Guide for People with Cancer and Their Families* and *Breakthrough Cancer Pain: Questions and Answers*. More information is also available on the Web at www.cancer.org.

PROSTHESES

Prostheses are human-made substitutes for missing body parts. Sometimes parts of the body must be removed if they contain cancer that could grow and spread. Prostheses are used to help a person look as though the body part had never been removed and to help the person function as normally as possible.

There are many different types of prostheses. Some are external, meaning they are worn on the outside and can be put on and taken off, while others are implanted during surgery. The prostheses most commonly needed by people with cancer are breast, leg, or testicular prostheses and penile implants. Wigs used to cover the temporary hair loss that may occur with some kinds of chemotherapy can also be considered prostheses.

WHAT THE PATIENT CAN DO

▶ Before surgery, ask your doctor about prostheses. Find out if you might need one and if the prosthesis can be applied or implanted during surgery. (Prostheses for testicles, breasts, and some limbs may be implanted during the first surgery.)

▶ Make sure you get a prescription for the prosthesis from your doctor because it may be covered by medical insurance.

For Patients Considering a Breast Prosthesis

▶ Contact your local chapter of Reach to Recovery®, a support group for women with breast cancer, for information and ideas. Call 800-ACS-2345 for information on resources in your area.

- If it makes you feel more comfortable, you can wear an external prosthesis while waiting for reconstructive surgery.

- Small prostheses (equalizers) are available for women who have had part of a breast removed in a lumpectomy or a segmental mastectomy.

- Nipple prostheses are available for breast reconstruction when the nipple cannot be saved. External nipple prostheses are also sold to cover flat or replace missing nipples.

- External prostheses, called breast forms, are sold in surgical supply stores, lingerie shops, and in the lingerie departments of many department stores. Call before you go to make sure that a professional fitter will be available.

- Have your partner or a good friend go with you, and don't hesitate to shop around to find the best fit and right price. Try many different types. Prostheses vary in shape, weight, and consistency. Custom-made forms are also available.

- Wear a form-fitting top when you shop for a prosthesis so that you can better see how it looks when you move. Prostheses may feel heavy, but they should feel comfortable, show natural contour and consistency, and remain in place when you move. Ask if the prosthesis absorbs perspiration, and find out how to care for it.

- Talk with your partner about your feelings about reconstructive surgery and changes in your body. See the section on sexuality on page 96 for more information.

For Patients Considering a Leg or Limb Prosthesis

- Ask before surgery about your options, including when and how your prosthesis will be fitted.

- Often a temporary leg prosthesis is fitted during the first surgery. Put your weight on it as advised by your doctor or physical therapist. The permanent prosthesis can be fitted after you are stronger.

- Cosmetic, nonfunctional limbs are available for people who cannot use a permanent prosthesis.

- Ask questions about how to care for the surgical site and the prosthesis. If you have discomfort, redness, or blisters, talk with your doctor. If the prosthesis needs adjustment, take it back to the prosthetist (the person who made and fit it) rather than trying to do it yourself.

For Patients Considering a Testicular Prosthesis

- A gel-filled plastic sac can be placed in the body during surgery or at a later date.

- Not all men want or feel that they need a testicular prosthesis. Discuss the possibility of a prosthesis with your partner.

- Talk with your doctor before surgery about whether you want a testicular prosthesis.

- See page 96 for more information about sexual relations after cancer treatment.

For Patients Considering a Penile Implant

- Penile implants or prostheses are typically placed in the body six to twelve months after surgery.

- Two different types of implants are available: inflatable and semi-rigid rod. Discuss the type that is best for you with your partner and your doctor. See page 96 for more information about sexual relations after cancer treatment.

 CALL THE DOCTOR if the patient develops redness, swelling, pain, pus, or drainage at the prosthesis site.

Radiation Therapy

Radiation therapy (or radiotherapy) uses an invisible ray or beam of high-energy particles to kill cancer cells. It is aimed at the cancer area, which is marked on the skin so that the beam is directed only to the cancer site. Sometimes small radioactive pellets, ribbons, or wires may be put into the tumor. Radiation can shrink tumors and relieve symptoms. Some cancers (such as Hodgkin disease) can be cured with radiation treatment. Other cancers (such as breast cancer) can now be treated with radiation to allow for less surgery.

Doctors do not expose people who are not ill to radiation treatment because it could cause problems for some. However, the benefit to people with cancer far outweighs the small risk of new problems. In order not to expose the people you care about to radiation, friends and relatives cannot be with you during the treatment itself. During external beam radiation treatments, you will be in a radiation therapy room by yourself. Technologists will watch you on a television monitor in a room close by and can hear you if you need anything during the actual treatment.

The side effects of radiation depend on the area of the body to be treated. Because radiation treats only a certain area of the body, its side effects tend to involve only that area. It is common during treatment for the skin to get red in the radiated area. It usually stays that way for three or four weeks after radiation treatments are completed. The skin may dry and flake or peel and ooze like a burn. Afterward, the skin may look darker or more tan for a few months or even for years.

With today's modern equipment and the skilled aiming of beams or careful placement of pellets or wires, the radiation dose is focused on the tumor. That way, other areas of the body do not suffer so many ill effects. For instance, if the chest is treated, there is no loss of scalp hair and usually no nausea or vomiting. On the other hand, if the brain requires treatment, hair loss is expected, and nausea and vomiting may occur because there is a "nausea center" in the brain. Talk with the radiation oncologist (the doctor trained to give radiation therapy) or oncology nurse about expected side effects.

WHAT THE PATIENT CAN DO

▸ Tell your doctor about all the medicines you are taking, including all over-the-counter medications or supplements, such as vitamins and herbs.

▸ Go to every scheduled therapy appointment.

▸ Ask questions. Your radiation treatment team is there to help you.

▸ If you suffer from nausea, vomiting, loss of appetite, diarrhea, or fatigue, tell your doctor or nurse and see the related sections in this book for suggestions on coping with these side effects.

▸ Sometimes small permanent markings are made before radiation therapy and sometimes ink is used to mark the area to receive therapy. If the area to be treated is marked on your skin in ink, ask your radiation team whether and when you can wash off the ink. You may need to take sponge baths instead of regular baths or showers to keep the markings in place.

▸ Protect the treated area from direct sunlight during treatment and for at least one year after treatment.

▸ Wear loose, comfortable clothing over the radiated area. Soft cotton clothing is preferred.

▸ Talk with the nurse or doctor about using skin creams, powder, deodorant, or makeup on the radiated skin. Avoid adhesive tape, hot or cold packs, and anything that dries or irritates skin.

▸ Bathe in lukewarm water using mild soap.

- Avoid crowds and don't visit with people who have colds, infections, coughs, or fevers.

- See "Blood Counts" on page 7 if hemoglobin, platelet, or white blood cell counts are low.

- Use birth control during radiation treatment and for three months afterward. (See page 96 for more information.)

- If the area that is being treated is in the pelvis (such as the bladder, prostate, vagina, cervix, or uterus), talk with your doctor or nurse about sexual side effects and what you can do. (See the section on sexuality on page 96.)

- If you notice skin blisters or oozing, talk to your doctor or nurse. You may need special dressings to protect the skin where you received radiation.

WHAT CAREGIVERS CAN DO

- Watch for fatigue, which may increase in the patient as cancer treatment continues. See page 42 for more on fatigue and ways in which the patient may need support.

- Encourage the patient to eat nutritious foods and drink enough liquids. The patient may need help preparing meals, especially later in treatment.

- Help the patient keep all appointments. Radiation treatment is often given every day for many weeks. You may need to get friends to drive the patient.

- Request that friends with infections visit only by phone until they are completely well.

- If the patient develops side effects or other symptoms, see the related sections in this book.

CALL THE DOCTOR if the patient has any of these symptoms:

- Bloody, weeping (wet), or discolored skin
- Fever of 100.5°F or higher, for temperature taken by mouth
- Pain

For more in-depth information, contact the American Cancer Society at 800-ACS-2345 and ask for *Understanding Radiation Therapy: A Guide for Patients and Families*. More information is also available on the Web at www.cancer.org.

Seizures

A seizure is the uncontrolled movement of muscles. It happens when nerve cells in the brain become overexcited and do not work properly. Seizures usually last less than five minutes. They are followed by a period of sleepiness and confusion, which can last for several hours. Seizures in cancer patients can be caused by high fevers, head injuries, serious infections of the fluid around the spine and brain, an imbalance in body chemistry, or tumor growth in the spine or brain. If the patient has a seizure, the eyes will stare blankly or roll back, and the body may jerk uncontrollably, especially the arms and the legs. The patient may lose control of the bladder and bowels.

WHAT THE PATIENT CAN DO

▸ Talk to the doctor about your seizures. Bring the person who saw your seizure to the doctor with you to answer the doctor's questions about it.

▸ Take anti-seizure medicines as prescribed.

WHAT CAREGIVERS CAN DO

▸ Stay calm. Try to notice what type of movements the patient makes, how long the seizure lasts, and what parts of the body move with the seizure.

▸ Stay with the patient and try to keep him or her safe. If a seizure occurs while the patient is in bed or on a chair, cradle the patient in your arms to keep him or her from falling to the floor.

▸ Loosen any clothing around the patient's neck.

▸ If the patient falls to the floor, place padding (e.g., rolled clothing) underneath the patient's head and roll the patient onto his or her left side.

- If the patient is lying on his or her back, gently turn the head to the side if possible. Do not move any part of the body forcefully.

- Avoid trying to open the patient's mouth during a seizure, even if the patient is biting his or her tongue. Keep fingers and hands away from the patient's mouth.

- Avoid moving the patient unless he or she is in a dangerous location (for instance, near a hot radiator, a glass door, or a stairwell).

- Once the seizure is over, cover the patient with a blanket and allow him or her to rest.

- Avoid giving the patient medicine, food, or liquid until the doctor is called and the patient is fully awake.

- If the patient is prone to seizures, use side rails and bumper pads on the bed. Be sure someone is with the patient when he or she is walking or sitting in a chair.

- Give anti-seizure medicine as prescribed by the doctor.

CALL THE DOCTOR if the patient has a seizure, once it is over and the patient is comfortable. If someone else is with you, stay with the patient and have the other person call the doctor.

Sexuality

Sexuality includes all the feelings and actions associated with loving someone. It includes holding hands, special looks, hugging, and kissing. It is not just the act of sex. This section addresses the side effects of different treatments that may affect your sex life and ways to relieve some common problems. Talk with your doctor or nurse and especially with your partner about any questions or concerns you may have. Remember that warmth, caring, physical closeness, and emotional intimacy are as necessary and rewarding as any other kind of human interaction.

Cancer treatment often affects the ability of men or women to have children. Chemotherapy, radiation, and some surgery can affect the reproductive system and cause infertility. In women, treatment may cause early menopause. It is hard to predict the outcome for any one person. Some people are still fertile after treatment; others are not.

Chemotherapy and radiation can also cause birth defects if a child is conceived during the course of treatment or within several weeks of ending treatment. Avoid pregnancy during chemotherapy or radiation therapy. Find out if there is a period of time you should wait after your specific type of treatment before trying to conceive. *Before treatment begins*, talk with your doctor about what to expect and about any plans to have children.

WHAT THE PATIENT CAN DO

▸ Realize that your sexual desire may decrease because of fears about your illness and treatment, as well as the treatment itself. For example, chemotherapy can make you very tired or sick. Radiation therapy to the pelvis or genital area can sometimes cause pain during sex.

Hormone treatment, removal of ovaries, or removal of testicles will change your body's hormone levels, which can affect sexual desire.

▸ Talk with your partner about your feelings and concerns.

▸ Wait until you feel ready for sexual activity. Do not push yourself.

▸ Express your desire for sexual contact when you feel able; do not wait for your partner to ask.

▸ If your white blood count is dangerously low, avoid intercourse to reduce your chance of infection. (See the section "Blood Counts" on page 7 for more information.) Ask your doctor whether this is an issue for you.

▸ Enjoy other forms of closeness, such as touching, caressing, and holding each other.

▸ If you've had radical surgery that has affected how you feel about yourself, ask your doctor if implants and/or reconstructive surgery are possible.

▸ Understand that you are not contaminated. You cannot give your partner cancer, and you cannot pass chemotherapy or radiation to your partner.

▸ Try other things if your usual sexual activities are uncomfortable. For example, you and your partner can use your hands to manually stimulate each other, or try oral–genital stimulation. Try caressing, fondling, and kissing each other. You can also try different positions that allow you to control thrusting, avoid pressure on tender areas, or avoid tiring (for example, lying on your sides facing each other, spooning, or switching who is on top).

Notes for men:

▸ Before you have chemotherapy or radiation to the genital area, ask your doctor about placing sperm in a sperm bank.

▸ In about forty to sixty percent of men, some degree of impotence (inability to get an erection) may develop gradually one or more years after radiation to the genital area. Impotence usually does not happen right after radiation treatment. This is different from the effects of prostate surgery, which are seen right away and may improve over time.

- Men who have been treated for testicular, prostate, bladder, colorectal, and even head and neck cancers often report having trouble getting erections after treatment.

- If you should have trouble getting an erection, ask your doctor about having your serum testosterone levels checked to determine whether hormone replacement therapy would help you. Ask about other medicines or treatments that may help you.

- Use erotic stimulation such as romantic dinners and prolonged foreplay.

- Shower together and use sexual play.

- Radiation treatment to the genital area can cause pain during ejaculation for a short time. It can also reduce the amount of semen and cause skin irritation.

- Men who have testicular cancer and have lymph nodes removed often have little or no semen at orgasm (called dry ejaculation). Return of semen may take months or years or may not happen at all. Semen is not needed for your or your partner's satisfaction.

- For men who have prostate cancer, blood in the semen is not unusual during diagnosis or treatment, especially after a needle biopsy. This is not harmful or worrisome but should be reported to your doctor.

- Urination may occur accidentally during sexual activity. There is no need for concern about this. Urine is normally sterile and will not harm your partner.

- Men with prostate cancer who have had radiation seeds implanted may need to use condoms for a few weeks, as the seeds may become dislodged during sexual activity. Ask your doctor how long you will need to use condoms.

Notes for women:

▶ Pain during intercourse is very common after surgery for many gynecologic cancers because the treatment may shorten or narrow the vagina. Ask your surgeon about the exact extent of your surgery. To help with pain during intercourse following treatment, try these techniques:

- Use sexual positions that give you control of the depth and force of thrusting (for example, try being on top or having both you and your partner lie on your sides).

- Use your thumb and index finger at the vaginal entrance to circle around the penis. This can provide extra length and keep your partner from thrusting too deeply.

- You can use techniques to keep the vagina from shrinking and tightening during radiation therapy to the pelvis or vagina. You will need to insert fingers, your partner's penis, or special vaginal dilators (enlargers) three to four times a week during the period in which you are receiving radiation treatment and for some time afterward.

- If surgery that involves the vagina is planned, talk with your doctor or nurse about vaginal dilators to use after surgery. Be sure to find out when to start and how to use them.

- Use an unscented, uncolored lubricant such as K-Y Jelly or Astroglide if lubrication becomes a problem. Surgery, radiation, or hormone treatment can cause dryness.

- Show your partner ways of touching you or positions that are comfortable to you. Before you try sex with your partner, check for soreness in your genital area.

▶ Chemotherapy can cause thinning of the vaginal wall. Slight bleeding after intercourse is not a major concern, but it may be alleviated by using extra water-based lubricant. Avoid contraceptive gels or foams, which contain a detergent that can irritate the vagina.

- Chemotherapy can also reduce sexual desire and make it harder to reach orgasm. This side effect usually gets better after treatment is over.

- Burning during intercourse may suggest a yeast infection. Talk to your doctor if you experience this symptom.

- Chemotherapy may cause you to stop menstruating for some time but may not entirely stop the ovaries from working. It may still be possible to get pregnant even if you haven't menstruated for several months. Talk with your doctor about birth control, since chemotherapy drugs can hurt a growing fetus.

- Chemotherapy, radiation, or surgery to remove the ovaries may cause early menopause. Ask your doctor about the chances of this happening in your situation.

- If infertility is likely, talk with your doctor about the possibility of freezing ovarian tissue or eggs. This does require special surgery and is very expensive, but this procedure may be an option for some women.

If you have an ostomy, try the following suggestions:

- Empty the pouch before sexual activity.

- Ask your enterostomal therapist about a pouch cover that doesn't look so "medical."

- If a leak occurs, shower together and continue sexual play.

- Tuck the pouch into a supportive belt.

- Turn the appliance to the side.

- Try different positions if there is friction.

- For women, crotchless, lacy underwear covers the appliance, but leaves the genital area open.

- Some people are more comfortable wearing a t-shirt to cover the stoma at first.

WHAT PARTNERS CAN DO

- Find out how cancer and cancer treatment are likely to affect your partner and your sexual relationship.

Chemotherapy can cause side effects and fatigue. Surgery and radiation in the genital area may permanently change the structure and functioning of the genitals.

- Learn what changes to expect if the person is taking hormones, which may affect sexual function or desire.

- Be patient during chemotherapy or radiation. Wait for times when your partner feels ready for sexual activity.

- Offer physical closeness and touching when the patient's energy is low. Intimacy can be achieved without intercourse, erections, or orgasms. Kindness, affection, and respect go a long way.

- Find out how the patient is feeling about his or her body and about sexual activity. Sometimes people feel unattractive after cancer treatment.

- It is normal to grieve losses and changes in body image, which affect both of you. Consider talking with a mental health professional if you have had difficult changes in your relationship.

- When your partner is ready, be willing to try more gentle activities and new positions that feel good to both of you. Plan for private time when you will not be interrupted.

- Use unscented, uncolored water-based lubricant (such as K-Y Jelly or Astroglide) if dryness causes discomfort for either of you.

- If you are afraid of hurting your partner, talk about it with your partner and with the doctor or nurse.

CALL THE DOCTOR if the patient has any of these symptoms:

- New or more severe pain
- Bleeding
- Change in erectile function or amount of semen
- Sexual problems or questions concerning sexual activity

For more in-depth information, contact the American Cancer Society at 800-ACS-2345 and ask for *Sexuality and Cancer: For the Woman Who Has Cancer and Her Partner* or *Sexuality and Cancer: For the Man Who Has Cancer and His Partner*. More information is also available on the Web at www.cancer.org. For questions about fertility options, such as freezing eggs or sperm before chemotherapy, visit www.fertilehope.org or call 888-994-HOPE.

Shortness of Breath

Trouble with breathing happens when the body is not getting enough oxygen. Either the lungs cannot take in enough air or the body cannot get enough oxygen through the bloodstream.

A number of different problems can cause shortness of breath, including chronic lung disorders, blocked airways, pneumonia, weak breathing muscles, or obesity. It can also be caused by pain, immobility, poor nutrition, stress or anxiety, allergic reactions, surgery, anemia, the side effects of chemotherapy or radiation treatment, a tumor, fluid in the lungs, heart failure, and other problems. The patient may have trouble breathing either at rest or with exercise. He or she may experience chest pain, quickened heartbeat, wheezing, or cold and clammy skin. Watch for pale or bluish skin, a blue color to the patient's fingernail beds, or flaring nostrils when the patient inhales.

WHAT THE PATIENT CAN DO

▶ If you are having trouble breathing, remain calm. Sit up or raise the upper body to a forty-five–degree angle by raising the bed or using pillows.

▶ Take any medicine or treatment prescribed for breathing, such as oxygen, medicine for relief of wheezing, inhalers, or nebulizers.

▶ If you are not in a lot of distress, check your temperature and pulse.

▶ Inhale deeply through your nose and exhale through pursed lips for twice as long as it took to inhale. This technique is called pursed-lip breathing.

- If you still feel no relief after five minutes, sit up on the side of the bed with your feet resting on a stool, your arms resting on an over-bed table or side table with pillows on it, and your head tilted slightly forward.

- If you are coughing and spitting, note the amount of sputum and what it looks and smells like.

- Talk with your doctor about how your breathing problem affects you, especially if you avoid some of your usual activities to keep from getting out of breath.

- Try muscle relaxation to reduce anxiety. Anxiety makes breathing problems worse.

- If you continue to have trouble breathing, ask your doctor about medicines you can use to make it easier to breathe.

- If new breathing problems start suddenly and do not improve, your skin looks pale or blue, or if you have chest discomfort, trouble speaking, dizziness, or weakness, get emergency help.

WHAT CAREGIVERS CAN DO

- Note the circumstances under which the patient gets out of breath. Does it happen when the patient is standing, sitting, or lying down? Is he or she typically doing strenuous activity, normal activity, or no activity?

- Check the patient's temperature to see if he or she has a fever.

- If the patient is short of breath, remove or loosen any tight clothing. Have the patient sit up in a resting position that feels comfortable to him or her. Remind him or her to take slow, deep breaths and exhale slowly.

- Remove the patient from extreme temperatures, especially heat, which may make it harder to breathe. Put the patient in front of an open window or a fan that blows gently on the face.

- Offer the patient any medicines or inhalers prescribed for shortness of breath.

▶ If home oxygen is prescribed, be sure you know how to set it up and what flow rate to use. Do not change the flow rate without first talking to the doctor. Don't allow smoking or fire when oxygen is in use.

CALL THE DOCTOR if the patient has any of these symptoms:

- Trouble breathing or chest pain
- Thick, yellow, green, and/or bloody sputum
- Pale or bluish skin or cold, clammy skin
- Fever of 100.5°F or higher, for temperature taken by mouth
- Flared nostrils during breathing
- Confusion or restlessness
- Trouble speaking
- Dizziness or weakness
- Swelling of the face, neck, or arms
- Wheezing

Skin Color Changes

Skin color changes usually happen because there is some type of change in the body. For example, a person may look yellow because of liver problems, blue because of breathing problems, bruised because of blood disorders, or red because of skin problems. Changes in the skin can be due to tumor growth, sun exposure, or side effects of chemotherapy or radiation therapy.

Some color changes may improve over time, while others may be permanent. The patient may see bruises or areas of blue or purple skin, redness or rash on the skin, deep orange urine, or white or clay-colored stools. There may be swelling in discolored areas, and the patient may also notice itching or difficulty breathing. Watch for yellowing in the skin or whites of the eyes.

WHAT THE PATIENT CAN DO

▸ Clean affected areas gently with warm water, gentle soap, and a soft cloth. Rinse the area carefully and pat dry. Apply a water-repellent cream, such as A&D Ointment.

▸ Wear loose-fitting clothing made of soft fabrics, such as cotton.

▸ Expose the affected skin to air whenever possible.

▸ Protect the affected area from heat and cold.

▸ Keep the skin protected from the sun. For instance, wear a wide-brimmed hat and long-sleeved shirts when outside.

▸ Apply sunscreen (SPF 15 and higher) to any skin exposed to sun.

▸ Apply medicine prescribed for skin reactions.

WHAT CAREGIVERS CAN DO

▸ Keep track of any new medicines, soaps, detergents, or foods in case they cause rashes or skin irritation on the patient.

▸ If the patient's hands are affected, do not let the patient do tasks involving hot water.

▸ Offer the patient gentle massages with moisturizing lotions or creams.

CALL THE DOCTOR if the patient has any of these symptoms:

- Urine that remains dark or orange for one day or more

- Stool that appears white or clay-colored for two or more bowel movements

- A yellowish color on the skin or in whites of the eyes

- Severe itching (See "Itching" on page 66.)

- Bruises that do not go away within one week, or if new bruises continue to appear for three days

- Red or rash-like areas on the skin

Skin Dryness

Dry skin can be rough, flaky, red, and sometimes painful. It is caused by low levels of oil and water in the layers of the skin. The skin may crack, and there can be slight bleeding in areas like the knuckles or elbows. Common causes of dry skin include dehydration, heat, cold, poor nutrition, and side effects of radiation treatment or chemotherapy.

WHAT THE PATIENT CAN DO

- Add mineral or baby oil to warm bath water or apply it after showering while skin is still damp. The oil can be slippery if it gets on surfaces, so be careful to keep from falling.
- Avoid scrubbing during showers or baths. Gently pat skin dry after bathing.
- Apply water-based creams twice a day, especially after baths.
- Avoid colognes, aftershaves, and after-bath splashes that contain alcohol.
- Use an electric razor for shaving rather than a blade.
- Drink two to three quarts of liquid a day, with approval from your doctor.
- Protect your skin from cold and wind. Avoid hot water and heat, especially dry heat.

WHAT CAREGIVERS CAN DO

- Apply lotions or oils on hard-to-reach places.
- Offer the patient extra fluids.

 CALL THE DOCTOR if the patient develops very rough, red, or painful skin, or if he or she has any signs of infection such as pus or tenderness near broken skin.

Skin Sores
(Pressure Sores)

A skin or pressure sore develops when the blood supply to an area of the body is stopped and the skin in that area dies. If a person is bedridden or always in a wheelchair, pressure is put on the same parts of the body for extended periods, reducing the blood flow to those places and making them more likely to develop sores. These areas are made worse when the patient rubs against his or her sheets or is pulled up roughly in the bed or chair. The sores may appear as red areas on the skin that do not go away even after the pressure is removed. The patient may have painful or tender "pressure points" on the back of the head, back of shoulders, elbows, buttocks, hips, heels, or any place a bony part rests on the bed surface. The skin may crack and blister, and the patient can develop open sores involving the skin surface or tissue under the skin. You may see yellowish or blood-tinged stains on clothing, bed sheets, or the patient's chair.

WHAT THE PATIENT CAN DO

▸ Change position at least every two hours, moving from your left side to your back then to your right side.

▸ If you are in a wheelchair, shift your weight every fifteen minutes. Use a special seat cushion to reduce pressure.

▸ Protect other pressure points with pillows to help prevent new sores. If possible, use a pressure-reducing mattress or a three- to four-inch foam layer over your mattress.

▸ Exercise as much as possible. If you can, take a short walk two or three times a day. If you are unable to walk, sit up and move your arms and legs up and down and back and forth.

- Eat foods that are high in protein, such as tuna or other fish, milk, and peanut butter.
- Increase fluids. (If you are not eating well, try high-calorie liquids such as milk shakes.)
- Bathe each day and monitor the pressure point areas.
- Always protect the sore and the area around it with a foam wedge or pillow.
- Rinse any open sore with water very carefully and cover with a clean bandage every time the bandage gets soiled or at least twice a day as instructed by your doctor or nurse. If your doctor gives you ointments or creams, use as prescribed. Report any itching or blistering in the area.

WHAT CAREGIVERS CAN DO

- Remind or help the patient to change position at least every two hours.
- If the patient cannot control his or her bowels and bladder, change the patient's underwear as soon as you notice soiling and then apply an ointment (such as A&D) to keep the area dry. Sprinkle cornstarch over the ointment. Avoid using plastic underwear unless the patient is out of bed. Use underpads to prevent soiling the bed while the patient is lying down.
- If the skin is open, talk with the doctor about special dressings to help protect it.
- If patient is bedridden, keep the bottom sheets pulled tight to prevent wrinkles and keep the head of the bed flat or at a thirty-degree angle. Sprinkle the sheets with cornstarch to reduce friction from rubbing against sheets.
- Inspect the patient's back and sides each day to be sure that the skin looks normal. If you notice any reddened "pressure areas," keep the pressure off as much as possible to try and prevent further breakdown. Use pillows and frequent position changes.

- If the patient has trouble staying on his or her side, consider using foam wedges to help the patient hold positions.

- Foam pads for beds and chairs may be helpful for some patients.

- If the patient continues to have problems with pressure sores, talk to the doctor or nurse about home care options. Find out about special beds that reduce pressure areas.

CALL THE DOCTOR if the patient has cracked, blistered, scaly, broken skin, a sore that is getting larger, a thick or bad-smelling liquid draining from the sore, or if the patient needs a referral to a home care agency for help with pressure sore care and supplies.

SLEEP PROBLEMS

Sleep problems can be defined as any change in the patient's usual sleeping habits. People who are getting treatment for cancer may get tired more easily and may need to sleep more than usual. Sometimes the opposite problem occurs and people may have trouble sleeping. Reasons for changes in usual sleeping habits include pain, anxiety, worry, and depression. Night sweats, side effects of treatment, or prescription drugs can also affect sleep.

WHAT THE PATIENT CAN DO

▶ Sleep as much as your body tells you to, but try to exercise at least once a day. You should do any exercise at least two to three hours before bedtime. (See the section on exercise on page 37.)

▶ Avoid drinks with caffeine for six to eight hours before bedtime.

▶ Avoid alcoholic drinks in the late evening. They can keep you awake as they "wear off."

▶ Drink warm, caffeine-free drinks, such as warm milk with honey or decaffeinated tea, before going to bed.

▶ Ensure a quiet setting for rest during the same period of time each day.

▶ Take sleeping medicine or pain relievers prescribed by the doctor at the same time each night. If pain keeps you awake, see the section on pain on page 82.

▶ Have someone give you backrubs or massage your feet before bedtime.

▶ Keep sheets clean, neatly tucked in, and as free from wrinkles as possible.

▶ Talk with your doctor about relaxation therapy or referral to a hypnotherapist.

WHAT CAREGIVERS CAN DO

▸ Help keep the room as quiet and comfortable as possible during the patient's sleep times.

▸ Offer the patient gentle backrubs or foot massages near bedtime.

▸ Offer the patient a light bedtime snack.

 CALL THE DOCTOR if the patient is confused at night or is unable to sleep at all during the night.

Steroids and Hormones

Hormones are natural substances in the body. Cortico-steroids (or steroids), such as cortisol, are produced by a small gland on top of each kidney. Estrogens are female hormones produced by the ovaries. Androgens, such as testosterone, are male hormones produced by the testes. Hormones and steroids can have an effect on different types of cancer, so some cancer treatments use steroids and hormones or hormone-blocking medications.

Testosterone can promote the growth of prostate cancer. That is why men with prostate cancer may take antiandrogen drugs to slow cancer growth. Estrogens are rarely used to treat prostate cancer.

Some breast cancers depend on estrogen to grow. Drugs that block estrogen or reduce its production, such as tamoxifen or aromatase inhibitors, are used to slow the growth of these types of breast cancer or keep them from coming back.

Corticosteroids are used to treat many different kinds of cancer. They also help to reduce nausea, improve appetite, and reduce swelling caused by cancer in the brain.

As with any treatment, taking corticosteroids, hormones, or hormone-blocking medications can cause side effects. It is important to watch for side effects so that you can talk to your doctor or nurse about ways to deal with them.

Estrogens can cause short-term side effects. In women, estrogens can cause fluid retention and vaginal discharge or bleeding. In men, they can cause tenderness and swelling of the breasts and less interest in sex. Estrogen-blocking drugs, such as tamoxifen, can cause hot flashes and vaginal dryness and discharge in women.

Androgen-blocking drugs may cause hot flashes in men, as well as a lowered interest in sex, decreased sexual performance, tiredness, and mood changes.

Corticosteroids can cause the following temporary side effects:

- Mood changes
- Trouble sleeping
- Fluid retention
- More facial hair
- Increased urination
- Increased thirst and appetite
- Muscle weakness
- Fat buildup in the cheeks, abdomen, and back of the neck.

Prolonged high doses of corticosteroids can cause osteoporosis (bone thinning), which raises the risk for broken bones.

WHAT THE PATIENT CAN DO

- Talk with your doctor about what to expect from your treatment.
- Limit your salt intake.
- Watch your calorie intake to avoid too much weight gain.
- Take your medicines as directed.
- Remember that these side effects are short-lived and will get better after the steroid or hormone treatment is done.
- Do not suddenly stop taking your medicines. Talk with your doctor if you experience any problems.

WHAT CAREGIVERS CAN DO

- Find out what medicines the patient is taking.
- Talk with the doctor so you will know what to expect while the patient is on hormone therapy.
- Watch for mood swings.

CALL THE DOCTOR if the patient has any of these symptoms:

- Vomiting or pain in the abdomen
- Disturbing mood swings
- Trouble sleeping
- Shortness of breath (See page 103 for more on shortness of breath.)
- Dehydration (See page 46 for more on fluids and dehydration.)
- Fever of 100.5°F or higher, for temperature taken by mouth
- Stools that look black like tar or contain blood
- Pain

For more in-depth information on the specific treatment you are receiving, contact the American Cancer Society at 800-ACS-2345 or on the Web at www.cancer.org.

STOMAS
(OSTOMIES)

A stoma is a surgically created opening in the body that replaces a normal opening. It is needed when the normal opening is blocked by tumor or has been removed as part of cancer treatment. Stomas serve as new sites for basic bodily functions. There are different types of stomas. Three commonly seen in people with cancer are a tracheostomy (pronounced tray-key-OSS-tuh-mee or "trake" for short) in the trachea (or windpipe), a urostomy in the bladder or urinary system, and a colostomy in the colon.

The following sections give more information on stomas and their care and maintenance.

Tracheostomy

WHAT THE PATIENT CAN DO

▸ Use a pad and paper for communicating with others.

▸ Do not remove the outer tube of the tracheostomy unless your doctor or nurse tells you to do so.

▸ Clean your tracheostomy tube at least once a day as instructed by your nurse or doctor.

▸ Suction the tube as needed or as directed by the nurse or doctor.

▸ Wash your hands carefully before and after handling your tracheostomy to help prevent infection.

▸ Be careful to keep water out of the stoma while bathing. A child's bib with the plastic side facing outward can be used to keep water out and allow breathing while you shower.

- Do not swim. Being around water that may reach your neck will be risky for you because water can get into your lungs.

- Wear a scarf or shirt that covers the opening but is made of a fabric (such as cotton) that allows air to get through. This helps protect the stoma from dust and loose fibers.

- Ask to meet with a respiratory therapist or ostomy nurse if you need more information.

- You may want to visit www.larynxlink.com or call 866-IAL-FORU to learn about the International Association of Laryngectomees.

Urostomy and Colostomy

WHAT THE PATIENT CAN DO

- Cleanse your skin gently every day with warm water only. (You may see a small amount of blood while cleansing. This is okay.)

- Gently pat your skin dry or allow to air dry.

- Showers or baths can be taken with pouch on or off.

- Apply barriers, borders, or pastes to the skin around the stoma before putting on the pouch.

- Empty the pouch when it is one-third full.

- Change your colostomy pouch before there is a leak—if possible, not more than once a day and not less than once every three or four days.

- Change your urostomy pouch every three to five days.

- Irrigate your stoma as instructed by a nurse or doctor.

- Ask your enterostomal therapy nurse or therapist any questions you may have.

- Consider joining a support group. Visit www.uoaa.org or call 800-826-0826 for information from United Ostomy Associations of America, Inc.

- See page 100 for tips on managing the stoma during sex.

WHAT CAREGIVERS CAN DO

▸ Learn how to care for the stoma, including the skin around the opening.

▸ If the patient has a tracheostomy, learn to suction out mucus from the upper airway. Moist air helps keep the patient's mucus from being too thick and sticky. A humidifier, especially in the bedroom, may be helpful. Check with the doctor or nurse on how to clean the humidifier.

▸ If the patient has a urostomy or colostomy, offer to help if the patient is having trouble. Often the patient feels embarrassed and will not ask for help.

▸ Encourage the patient to join an ostomy club for support and practical tips.

Swallowing Problems

Swallowing problems occur when a person has trouble getting foods or liquids down his or her throat. The person may gag, cough, vomit, or spit when trying to swallow. It may feel like the food is sticking on the way down, and there may be pain in the throat or mid-chest when he or she swallows. There can be a number of causes. It may be a short-term side effect of chemotherapy or radiation treatment to the throat or chest. It may also be caused by an infection of the mouth or esophagus (the swallowing tube that goes from the throat to the stomach) or by other problems.

The patient may have sores or white patches in the mouth, and the inside of the mouth may be red, shiny, or swollen. The patient could have either little saliva or too much saliva due to swallowing difficulties and may drool out of the side of the mouth. Swallowing problems also can lead to weight loss.

WHAT THE PATIENT CAN DO

▸ Eat bland foods that are soft and smooth but high in calories and protein (like pudding, gelatin, ice cream, yogurt, and milk shakes).

▸ Take small bites, and swallow each bite completely before taking another.

▸ Use a straw for liquids and soft foods.

▸ Try thicker liquids (such as fruit that has been puréed in the blender)—they are easier to swallow than thin liquids.

▸ Mash or purée foods (such as meats, cereals, and fresh fruits) so that they are as soft as baby food. You may need to add liquids to dry foods before blending.

- Dunk breads in milk to soften.

- Serve food cold (the cold helps numb pain) or cool. Pain in the esophagus may feel worse with cold liquids. If so, serve food at room temperature.

- Try crushed ice and liquids at meals.

- Frequent small meals and snacks may be easier to manage.

- Crush medicines in pill or tablet form; mix in to juice, applesauce, jelly, or pudding. Check with your nurse or pharmacist first, because some medicines can be dangerous if crushed or broken. Others react badly with certain foods; still others must be taken on an empty stomach.

- Avoid alcohol and hot, spicy foods or liquids.

- Avoid acidic foods, such as citrus fruits and drinks or fizzy sodas (like cola or ginger ale).

- Avoid hard, dry foods like crackers, nuts, and chips.

- Sit upright for eating and drinking and for a few minutes after meals.

- If pain is a problem, use a numbing gel or pain reliever such as viscous lidocaine (by doctor's prescription) or liquid Tylenol. (See "Mouth Sores" on page 75 for more about mouth pain.)

- Ask your doctor about seeing a speech therapist or swallowing therapist.

WHAT CAREGIVERS CAN DO

- Offer the patient soft, moist foods. Baked egg dishes, tuna salads, and thick liquids such as yogurt may be easier to swallow because of their texture.

- Help the patient avoid chewy foods or raw, crunchy vegetables.

- Offer the patient sauces and gravies that might make meats easier to swallow.

CALL THE DOCTOR if the patient has any of these symptoms:

- Increased gagging, coughing, or choking, especially while eating or drinking

- Severe sore throat

- Red, shiny mouth or ulcers in the mouth or on the tongue

- Fever of 100.5°F or higher, for temperature taken by mouth

- Trouble breathing

- Chest congestion

- Problems with food "sticking" as it goes down

- Inability to swallow medicines or eat

Sweating

Sweating is heavy perspiration. It can happen at night, even when the room is cool, and can be heavy enough to soak a person's clothing. The patient may feel wet or damp during the night or may wake to find the sheets damp. Such sweating is common when a fever breaks. You may notice sweating happening a short time after the person has shaking chills. (See "Fever" on page 44 for more information.) You can have a fever with or without a known infection. Sometimes no fever is detected, only the sweating that goes along with a drop or break in fever.

WHAT THE PATIENT CAN DO

▸ Take medicine such as Tylenol to reduce your fever if instructed by the doctor or nurse.

▸ Dress in two layers of clothing. The layer on the outside will act as a wick to pull moisture up and away from the skin.

▸ Change wet clothes as soon as possible.

▸ Keep bed linens dry.

▸ Bathe at least once a day to soothe skin and to maintain good hygiene.

WHAT CAREGIVERS CAN DO

▸ Help the patient keep clothes and bed linens dry.

▸ Check the patient's temperature several times to find out if there is fever.

▸ Offer the patient extra liquids to replace the fluid that is lost through sweating.

▸ For comfort, try to help with a tub bath or a shower if the patient is able.

CALL THE DOCTOR if the patient becomes dehydrated from frequent soaking sweats; has a fever of 100.5°F or higher, for temperature taken by mouth; or has tremors or shaking chills.

SWELLING

Swelling (edema) is a buildup of water in the tissues. Common causes include salt and water retention (due to medicines or because of heart, liver, or kidney failure), poor nutrition, pelvic tumors, or a blockage in the veins or lymphatic system. Fluid can also build up in the abdomen. This is known as ascites (pronounced uh-SIGH-tees). It makes the belly look swollen and puffy. Patients with swelling may notice that the feet and lower legs get larger when they sit, stand, or walk. Rings may feel too tight for the fingers, and the hands can feel tight when you make a fist. The patient may have trouble breathing, especially when lying down, and may notice the heart racing or palpitations.

WHAT THE PATIENT CAN DO

- Eat as well as you can. Limit the use of salt on your food. Avoid the use of table salt and salt in cooking, and don't eat foods that are very high in salt. Talk with the doctor about how to reduce your salt intake.
- Take medicines as prescribed by the doctor.
- Rest in bed with your feet up on two pillows.
- When sitting up in a chair, keep your feet level with your chest on a stool with pillows.

WHAT CAREGIVERS CAN DO

- Watch for any new symptoms, especially shortness of breath or swelling in the face.
- Encourage the patient to keep the swollen body part propped up as high as is comfortable when sitting or lying down.

- Don't add salt, soy sauce, or monosodium glutamate during cooking.

- Every day or two, weigh the patient on the same scale at the same time of day. Keep a list of weights and dates.

CALL THE DOCTOR if the patient has any of these symptoms:

- Inability to eat for a day or more

- Infrequent or no urination for a day or more

- Any swollen area where a finger pressed into the area leaves a fingertip mark

- Swelling that spreads up legs or arms

- Puffy or blown-up belly

- Swollen area that gets red or hot

- Shortness of breath or racing heart

- Swollen face and neck, especially in the mornings

- Weight gain of five or more pounds in a week or less

TREATMENT AT HOME

Treatment for cancer can sometimes be given at home rather than in a hospital or clinic. Pills, intravenous (IV) chemotherapy, IV antibiotics, subcutaneous injections (shots given under the skin, also known as sub-Q injections), intramuscular injections (shots given into a muscle, also known as IM injections), and other treatments may be given at home. Talk with your doctor about the option of home care. It is important to take medicines as prescribed and to watch for side effects. Usually, a home care nurse or IV therapy (infusion) nurse will make frequent visits to your home to give, teach you about, or check on home treatments.

Home treatments are sometimes not an option because of problems with health insurance. You may want to contact your insurance company to find out more. Patients who cannot make frequent visits to the doctor's office or clinic may qualify for some kinds of home care. This requires that you be homebound, only going out for doctor's visits or church.

WHAT THE PATIENT CAN DO

Pills

▶ Take your pills exactly as you were told.

▶ You may have to set an alarm and get up in the middle of the night to take your pills at the right time.

▶ If taking pills only once a day, you may want to try taking them just before bedtime to avoid side effects, such as nausea. Talk with your doctor or nurse about the best time and way to take each medicine.

- ▶ Ask your doctor or nurse about any side effects you may have and about ways to control them. For instance, if your pills could cause nausea, ask if you should take them before meals or if there is something else you can take that would help.

- ▶ Keep all medicines out of the reach of children and pets.

- ▶ Check with your doctor, nurse, or pharmacist before you cut or crush your pills. Some time-release drugs can be dangerous if the pills are broken.

Intravenous (IV) Medicine

- ▶ A home health care or infusion nurse may come to your home to give drugs intravenously (into a vein) or to teach you and your family how to give these.

- ▶ See "Tubes and Intravenous (IV) Lines" on page 131 for further information on care of the IV site.

Injections (Under the Skin or into a Muscle)

- ▶ Wash your hands well with soap and water before starting.

- ▶ Take your medicines as instructed by your doctor or nurse.

- ▶ Check to be sure that the dosage in the syringe is your prescribed dosage.

- ▶ Wipe the skin with alcohol and let it dry for thirty seconds before injecting.

- ▶ If the needle touches anything that isn't sterile before you inject, throw the needle away, put a new one on the syringe, and start over.

- ▶ Use a different place on the body for each injection.

- ▶ Use a site that is at least one inch away from the place you used before for shots under the skin.

- ▶ For intramuscular injections, ask for a picture or chart of places on the body that are safe to use.

- Check old injection sites for signs of infection: redness, warmth, swelling, pain, or oozing. An oral temperature of 100.5°F or higher may be a sign of infection.

- Put used needles and syringes in an empty coffee can with a lid or a plastic bleach bottle as soon as you're finished. Take the full container to the clinic for proper disposal. Or ask the home health nurse if you can get a needle disposal box. Keep the needle container away from children, pets, and visitors.

WHAT CAREGIVERS CAN DO

- Learn how to give any medicines in case the patient is unable to do it.

- If you help with injections, be careful not to stick yourself with the needles. Put the used needle container near the patient before you start. Drop the needle and syringe in as soon as you're finished. Don't put the cap back on the needle.

- Keep the doctor's office number (including emergency numbers) handy.

- If there is a home health care nurse who helps with injections, keep the agency number nearby in case you have questions.

- Keep all medications away from children and pets.

- Monitor the supply of medications to be sure the doctor is called for any necessary refills.

CALL THE DOCTOR if the patient has any of these symptoms:

- Redness, warmth, swelling, drainage, or pain at any injection site
- Fever of 100.5°F or higher, for temperature taken by mouth
- Uncomfortable side effects such as nausea, vomiting, diarrhea, or pain

Also, call the doctor if any of the following happens:

- The patient misses a dose or throws up a dose
- The patient spills or loses medicine
- The patient cannot give himself or herself the medication for any reason

CALL THE DOCTOR IMMEDIATELY if any person other than the patient takes any of his or her medication or if the patient develops itching, dizziness, shortness of breath, hives (raised itchy skin welts), or other signs of an allergic reaction after an injection. If the symptoms are severe, call 911 before calling the doctor.

TUBES AND INTRAVENOUS (IV) LINES

Tubes and intravenous (IV) lines allow liquid medicines, fluids, and even nourishment to flow into the body. See "Treatment at Home" on page 127 for more information.

With tube feedings, liquid food is given through a tube placed in the stomach or the small intestine. The tube may go in through the nose or the wall of the stomach. Oxygen can be given through a mask or little tubes called nasal cannulae, which are placed just inside the nostrils. Tubing connects the mask or cannula to the oxygen tank.

IV lines are thin, flexible, plastic hoses that run from a bottle or bag of medicine into a tiny needle or intravenous catheter (a small flexible tube) placed in a vein in your body. Some patients may have a port (like a small drum) permanently placed in the chest or arm. Special needles are then put into the port. Some patients may have long-term catheters that do not require needles.

Some medicines are injected into the catheter, while other medicines and fluids are given slowly (infused). The speed, or rate, of the infusion is set by a roller clamp on the tube, a balloon that squeezes out the medicine, or an electronic pump.

Nutrient solutions also can be given intravenously. This type of therapy is called hyperalimentation (also called total parenteral nutrition, or TPN).

An important difference between these types of tubes is that anything that goes in the IV line must be sterile (completely germ free), to avoid putting germs into the bloodstream and causing infections. IV equipment is used only once. It must be handled carefully to keep germs out of the body. After use, it is thrown out and replaced with new, sterile equipment fresh out of the package. Tube feedings and oxygen tubes are kept clean, but do not have to be sterile. Tube feeding or oxygen equipment can be reused as long as it is used by the same person. When tube feeding bags need cleaning, dish soap and water are sufficient.

People getting chemotherapy, antibiotics, hyperalimentation, tube feedings, and/or oxygen at home may be faced with many tubes and IV lines to keep track of and learn to use safely. At first it may seem confusing, but you can master taking care of many tubes or lines. A home health care nurse will help you learn. Usually, chemotherapy and blood products are given by a nurse who comes to your home. You and your family will be able to manage most other IV medicines. If you cannot, other plans will be made for you to get your treatment.

WHAT THE PATIENT CAN DO

IVs

▶ Focus on only one set of lines at a time. If you get frustrated, just take a deep breath and start again.

▶ Color code each set of lines with colored tape. For example, red for chemotherapy, green for antibiotics, etc. Keep a record of what you have marked. You may want to use blue tape on oxygen tubes to keep them clearly separate from the IV lines.

▶ For permanent IV sites (for example, Hickman, Port-a-Cath, PasPort, Infusaport), follow these important guidelines:

- Carry extra clamps at all times.

- If a tube breaks and you notice blood leaking out, clamp the tube between your body and the leak and call your doctor right away.

- Shower facing away from the shower head. If you have an electric pump, unplug it before showering or bathing to avoid electrical hazard. Try to keep the dressing dry, and change it if it gets wet.

- Watch for redness, swelling, pain, and tenderness at the site.
- Use a calendar to record when you change your injection caps and dressings and to note delivery dates, daily weights, and urine testing results. It is also helpful to record your daily fluid intake and output (how much liquid you drink and infuse and how much urine you put out). Your doctor or nurse should tell you what things you need to track.

▸ Keep your IV site clean and dry.

▸ Avoid the temptation to speed up your IV medicines or fluids. Many IV medicines and fluids can harm you if infused too fast.

▸ Wash your hands well with soap and water before touching the IV site.

▸ Check the IV site daily for the following things:

- Be sure that tape is holding the IV in place and the dressing is clean and dry.
- Look for any tenderness, pain, redness, burning, swelling, or warmth; any slowing of the flow rate of the IV; and any drainage (bloody, yellowish, or clear).
- If you notice any of the above symptoms, remove the dressing and inspect the site. Carefully apply a new dressing, and report the findings to your doctor.

▸ Check your temperature daily and report any fever of more than 100.5°F, for temperature taken by mouth, to your doctor.

▸ If the IV comes out or the site begins to bleed, call your doctor or nurse right away.

▸ Avoid activities that may pull out your IV or rub on the dressing.

▸ Keep a daily log of the procedures performed.

Hyperalimentation (TPN or Total Parenteral Nutrition)

▸ Your home health care nurse will teach you exactly how to begin and end each infusion.

▸ Infuse slowly overnight, so that you have more free time during the day.

▸ If you find that you are having trouble sleeping because you need to go to the bathroom often, TPN may be infused during the day or early evening. It still must be infused slowly.

▸ Intravenous fat emulsions are usually given along with TPN two to seven times a week to provide essential fatty acids and to increase calorie intake: the fat emulsions can be added to the TPN solution through a port on the TPN tubing. These can be infused by gravity (without a pump) in adults. Your home health care nurse will show you how to set the speed by using the roller clamp and timing it to give you the right number of drops per minute. A pump is needed for children.

▸ Infuse your TPN in a room near a bathroom so that you do not have to carry the pump too far. Use a night light so that if you need to get up at night, you don't trip over or pull the tubing.

▸ Most pumps are battery powered. Check with the home health care team about how long the pump can run before new batteries are needed. Be sure you have enough batteries for your type of pump and know how to put them in.

▸ Keep a clean work area for supplies.

▸ If possible, use a separate place in the refrigerator (or a separate refrigerator if you have an extra one) for IV solutions.

▸ Throw away needles and syringes in a metal coffee can with a lid, a bleach bottle, or in a container provided by the home health care team. Keep the container out of the reach of children, pets, and others.

- Always check the expiration date on all supplies.
- Home health care nurses will draw blood samples to check fluids and blood chemistry.

Tube Feedings

- Tubes may be short- or long-term. The nasogastric tube (sometimes called an NG tube), which runs from nose to stomach, is for short-term use. Jejunostomy tubes (J tubes) or gastrostomy tubes (G tubes), which are surgically placed in the upper intestine or stomach and come out through the belly, are for long-term use.
- Tube feedings are best given at night.
- Feedings usually consist of products like Ensure or Sustacal.
- Give tube feedings at room temperature. Most do not need to be refrigerated.
- Check the placement of nasogastric tubes as instructed by a doctor or nurse.
- Pour feeding liquid into the special feeding bag.
- Allow the feeding liquid to run through the entire tubing. Tap the tube to make air bubbles rise.
- Attach the tube containing the feeding liquid to the nasogastric tube, gastrostomy tube, or jejunostomy tube. Tape the connection.
- Set the pump to the required rate.
- Add more feeding liquid to the bag as needed.
- Rinse the tubes and the bag with water after the infusion is completed.
- Cap off the tube as instructed.
- Feedings can also be given with large syringes instead of bags and tubing. Be sure you are comfortable using whichever method you are taught.
- Check the skin around tubes each day for redness, drainage, or skin problems.

- Apply petroleum jelly (Vaseline) to the nostrils if a nasogastric tube is in place.

- Change the tape on the nasogastric tube every other day. Be sure the skin around the nose and nostrils is not sore, red, or painful.

- Weigh yourself each day and write down the dates and weights.

Oxygen

- Be sure you know how to turn the oxygen on and off and how to set the flow rate. Never increase the oxygen flow above the prescribed level.

- The nurse will show you how to use the oxygen mask or cannula.

- Use a water-based lubricant, rather than petroleum jelly, on the lips and cheeks.

- If the nasal cannula rubs your upper lip, you can put a small piece of gauze or fabric under it for padding.

- Keep a new tank of oxygen available at all times. Even if you use an oxygen machine, you will need a small tank for leaving the house or in the event of a power failure.

- If you use a tank, be sure it is attached to a stable cart so it won't fall or roll.

- Do not smoke or go near sparks or flames while using oxygen. Keep sparks and flames away from tanks, oxygen machines, and tubing.

WHAT CAREGIVERS CAN DO

- Learn as much as you can about how to use the tubes and equipment, and practice while the home health care nurse is there to watch you. You may need to do these tasks when the patient cannot.

- Help the patient. In the beginning, you will probably both feel more comfortable if you do these treatments together.

- Keep home health care nurses' phone numbers handy, and call when you have questions or problems.
- Be sure the patient keeps all appointments.
- Watch for confusion in the patient, especially at night.

CALL THE DOCTOR if the patient has any of these symptoms:

- Redness, swelling, drainage, pain, tenderness, or warmth at an IV site or at the site of a permanent IV access device
- Fever of 100.5°F or higher, for temperature taken by mouth
- Bleeding from the IV or access site
- Cannot flush or use his or her catheter or tube
- Change in mental status (for instance, if the patient becomes drowsy or confused)
- Increased shortness of breath
- Cough
- Diarrhea for more than one day

WEIGHT CHANGES

Weight changes during treatment for cancer are common. There are a number of causes for weight loss, including eating less because of nausea or poor appetite, diarrhea, vomiting, and dehydration. Causes for weight gain include decreased activity, eating more, retaining water, and certain medicines.

Any weight change of more than five pounds in a week should be reported to your doctor. A decrease in weight over time may affect one's ability to function, leaving people feeling weak and unable to perform daily activities. Quick weight loss is often a sign of dehydration, which also can be signaled by dry skin and extreme thirst.

An increase in weight over time may suggest a serious health condition, such as diabetes or high blood pressure. The patient may feel puffy or bloated, have swollen ankles, or feel short of breath.

You may be able to tell if you gain or lose five pounds in a week by the way you feel or the way your clothes fit, but it is best to weigh yourself on a scale regularly.

WHAT THE PATIENT CAN DO

▸ *If you have lost weight*, drink extra high-protein and high-calorie fluids between meals. Be sure to drink enough water or other liquids that have no caffeine. Eat high-protein foods. You may also try liquid food supplements. Ask your doctor or nurse to arrange a meeting with a dietitian.

▸ *If you have gained weight*, talk with your doctor or nurse about limiting fluid if your ankles are swollen. Limit salt intake and high-calorie foods, and ask your doctor or nurse to arrange a meeting with a dietitian.

WHAT CAREGIVERS CAN DO

▸ Weigh the patient at the same time every day and write it down along with the date. In the morning before breakfast is a good time.

▸ Talk to the doctor if the patient's weight loss or weight gain concerns you.

▸ Watch patient for other symptoms.

CALL THE DOCTOR if the patient has any of these symptoms:

- Weight change (loss or gain) of more than five pounds in one week

- Shortness of breath

- Dizziness or confusion

CONCLUSION

Through the information presented in this book, we have tried to prepare you for some of the problems and concerns you may face as a caregiver. We've also tried to make a few suggestions for coping with some of the stresses that may come with caring for the person with cancer at home. If you or your family would like more information, please call the American Cancer Society anytime, day or night, at 800-ACS-2345. We have cancer information specialists who can help you with your questions and help you find the resources you need.

REFERENCES

American Cancer Society. *American Cancer Society's Guide to Pain Control: Understanding and Managing Cancer Pain, Revised ed.* American Cancer Society: Atlanta, 2004.

American Society for Therapeutic Radiology and Oncology. *RT Answers— Answers to Your Radiation Therapy Questions.* http://www.rtanswers.org. Accessed November 30, 2006.

Anonymous. Nocturnal Leg Cramps. *Postgraduate Medicine Online.* 2002;3(2). http://www.postgradmed.com/issues/2002/02_02/pn_legcramps.shtml. Accessed March 20, 2008.

Braunwald E, Fauci AS, Kasper DL, et al (eds). *Harrison's Principles of Internal Medicine, 15th ed.* New York: McGraw-Hill, 2001.

Camp-Sorrell D, Hawkins RA. *Clinical Manual for the Oncology Advanced Practice Nurse, 2nd ed.* Pittsburg: Oncology Nursing Society, 2006.

Cope DG, Reb AM. *An Evidence-Based Approach to the Treatment and Care of the Older Adult with Cancer.* Pittsburgh: Oncology Nursing Society, 2006.

Houts PS, Bucher JA. *Caregiving, Revised ed.* Atlanta: American Cancer Society, 2003

Kaplan M. *Understanding and Managing Oncologic Emergencies: A Resource for Nurses.* Pittsburgh: Oncology Nursing Society, 2006.

Kuebler KK, Berry PH, Heidrich DE. *End-of-Life Care: Clinical Practice Guidelines.* Philadelphia: WB Saunders, 2002.

National Cancer Institute. *Gene Therapy for Cancer: Questions and Answers.* http://www.cancer.gov/cancertopics/factsheet/Therapy/gene. Accessed November 10, 2006.

National Comprehensive Cancer Network and the American Cancer Society. *Cancer-Related Fatigue and Anemia: Treatment Guidelines for Patients, Version II.* Atlanta, GA: American Cancer Society, 2003.

Oncology Nursing Society. *Symptoms.* http://www.cancersymptoms.org. Accessed November 30, 2006.

Ripamonti C, Bruera E. *Gastrointestinal Symptoms in Advanced Cancer Patients.* New York: Oxford University Press, 2002.

University of Kentucky Health Information Library. *Tracheostomy, Adult.* http://www. ukhealthcare.uky.edu/patiented/ed/Tracheostomy,%20Adult%20June%202003. pdf. Accessed March 20, 2008.

Varricchio CG. *A Cancer Source Book for Nurses, 8th ed.* Sudbury, MA: Jones and Bartlett, 2004.

Yarbro CH, Frogge MH, Goodman M. *Cancer Symptom Management, 3rd ed.* Sudbury, MA: Jones and Bartlett, 2004.

ADDITIONAL RESOURCES

More Information from the American Cancer Society

The following information may also be helpful to you. These free materials may be ordered from our toll-free number, 800-ACS-2345. More information is also available on the Web at www.cancer.org. Materials marked (**S**) are also available in Spanish.

Advanced Cancer and Palliative Care: Treatment Guidelines for Patients (**S**)

Advanced Directives

Advanced Illness: Financial Guidance for Cancer Survivors and Their Families

Anxiety, Fear, and Depression

Bone Metastasis

Breakthrough Cancer Pain: Questions and Answers

Cancer Pain: Treatment Guidelines for Patients (**S**)

Cancer-Related Fatigue and Anemia: Treatment Guidelines for Patients (**S**)

Clinical Trials: What You Need to Know

Coping with Grief and Loss (**S**)

Distress: Treatment Guidelines for Patients (**S**)

Family Medical Leave Act

Helping Children When a Family Member Has Cancer

Helping Children When a Family Member Has Cancer: Dealing with a Parent's Terminal Illness

Home Care Agencies (**S**)

Hospice Care (**S**)

Listen with Your Heart: Talking with the Person Who Has Cancer (**S**)

Medical Insurance and Financial Assistance for the Cancer Patient (**S**)

A Message of Hope: Coping with Cancer in Everyday Life (**S**)

Nausea and Vomiting: Treatment Guidelines for Patients with Cancer (**S**)

Nutrition for the Person with Cancer: A Guide for Patients and Families (**S**)

Pain Control: A Guide for People with Cancer and Their Families (**S**)

Sexuality and Cancer: For the Man Who Has Cancer and His Partner (**S**)

Sexuality and Cancer: For the Woman Who Has Cancer and Her Partner (**S**)

Talking with Friends and Relatives about Your Cancer (**S**)

Talking with Your Doctor (**S**)

Understanding Chemotherapy: A Guide for Patients and Families

Understanding Psychosocial Support Services

Understanding Radiation Therapy: A Guide for Patients and Families

Understanding Your Lab Values

INDEX

Consciousness, changes near death, 59–60

Confusion, 23–25
and blood in urine, 15
and dehydration, 47
and difficulty moving, 36
and fatigue, 43
and fever, 44, 45
and hemoglobin, low, 8
and immunotherapy, 65
and nausea and vomiting, 81
from pain medication, 84
and shortness of breath, 105
and violent behavior, 25
what the caregiver can do,
24–25, 137
what the patient can do, 23
when to call the doctor, 8, 15,
23, 25, 36, 43, 47, 81, 86, 105

Constipation, 26–27, 34, 84, 86

Coping, 1, 28

Corticosteroids, 114–116

Counseling, 1, 2, 3, 28, 29, 30, 101

Cramps
abdominal, 34
leg, 69–70
stomach, 17, 26, 27

D

Death
approach of, 57–63
body functions near, 58–59
breathing changes near, 62
circulation changes near, 61
consciousness changes near,
59–60
elimination changes near,
62–63
at home, 63
metabolism changes near, 60
perception changes near, 62
secretion changes near, 60–61
senses changes near, 62
signs of, 57–58
temperature changes near, 61

Dehydration, 46–47
avoiding, with fever, 45
and fatigue, 42
with frequent soaking sweats,
124
and loss of appetite, 4, 6
when to call the doctor, 6, 47,
116, 124

Dental care
with low platelet count, 11
with low white blood cell count,
10
and mouth bleeding, 71–72
and mouth dryness, 73–74
mouth rinse, gentle, 73, 76
and mouth sores, 75–78
mouthwashes, store-bought,
avoiding, 71, 73, 76
periodontal disease, 71
toothbrushing, 71, 75–76

Dentures, 72, 76

Depression, 28–31
and anxiety, 1, 28
drug therapy for, 29–30
symptoms of, 28–29
what the caregiver can do, 30
what the patient can do, 29–30
when to call the doctor, 29, 30,
31

Diarrhea, 32–34
and constipation, 26–27
and dehydration, 47
diet for, 32, 33
what the caregiver can do, 33
what the patient can do, 32–33
when to call the doctor, 17, 27,
34, 47, 130, 137

Difficulty moving, 35–36
when to call the doctor, 11

Disorientation. *See* Confusion

Dizziness
and allergic reaction, 130
and bleeding, 72
and dehydration, 46, 47
and exercise, 38
and falls, avoiding, 39

and hemoglobin, low, 8, 17
and hiccups, 55
and immunotherapy, 65
and nausea or vomiting, 81
and shortness of breath, 104, 105
weight change and, 139
when standing, 47
when to call the doctor, 8, 17,
38, 47, 65, 72, 81, 104, 105,
130, 139

E

F

CANCER CAREGIVING A TO Z

Nausea, 79–81. *See also* Vomiting
   and chemotherapy, 18, 19
   and constipation, 26
   and corticosteroids, 114
   and pain medicine, 84
   and poor appetite, 4
   and radiation therapy, 91
   severe, and immunotherapy, 65
   what the caregiver can do, 81
   what the patient can do, 79–80
   when to call the doctor, 6, 17,
      65, 81, 130

Night sweats, 112, 123

Nipple prostheses, 88

Nosebleeds, 11

Nurse, home health, 127, 128, 129,
   132, 136, 137

Nutrition
   to combat leg cramps, 70
   and constipation, 26, 27
   and diarrhea, 32–33
   and fatigue, 43
   and low blood cell counts, 8, 9
   with mouth sores, 77
   during nausea, 79–80
   and poor appetite, 4
   for weight changes, 138
   when eating is difficult, 120–121

Nutrition, total parenteral (TPN),
   134–135

O

Opioids, 82, 84, 85

Oral health. *See* Dental care; Mouth

Osteoporosis, 115

Ostomies, 117–119
   colostomy, 118, 119
   managing, during sex, 100
   tracheostomy, 117–118, 119
   urostomy, 118, 119

Oxygen, at home, 105, 131, 132, 136

P

Pain, 82–86
   breakthrough, 83, 85
   dosing errors, avoiding, 85
   and fatigue, 42
   medicine for controlling, 82–83,
      84, 85, 86
   and mouth sores, 75–76, 77
   and moving difficulties, 35
   pleasant events as distraction, 85
   and radiation therapy, 93
   during sex, 96, 97, 98, 99
   unrelieved, 84
   what the caregiver can do,
      84–85
   what the patient can do, 83–84
   when to call the doctor, 6, 8,
      15, 17, 20, 27, 34, 36, 38, 45,
      70, 86, 89, 93, 101, 105, 108,
      116, 130, 137

Pain specialist, consulting, 84

Palpitations, 43, 125, 126

Parenteral nutrition, total, 134–135

PasPort, 132

Perception, changes in, near death,
   61–62

Perspiration, 123–124

Permanents, hair, avoiding, 51

Pills, 127–128
   difficulty swallowing, 85, 121

Platelet count, 7, 10–11, 71

Port-a-Cath, 132

Pouches, ostomy, 118

Pregnancy, avoiding during therapy,
   19, 92, 96

Pressure sores, 12, 109–111

Prostheses, 87–89
   for breasts, 87–88
   for limbs, 88–89
   for nipples, 88
   penile implants, 89
   for testicles, 89
   when to call the doctor, 89

Speech, problems with, 11, 23, 104, 105

Speech, therapist for, swallowing difficulties, 121

Sputum, discolored, 104, 105

Stem cell transplants, 16–17

Steroids, 114–116

Stomas, 117–119

Stomatitis, 71–72, 75–78

Stool
color of, 8, 10, 13, 107, 116
near death, 62, 63
passing hard, 26
softeners, 26, 84, 85

Suicide, thoughts of, 29, 31

Sunscreen, use of, 51, 106

Supplements, 3, 5

Support groups, 30, 85, 118, 119

Sustacal, 5, 135

Swallowing problems, 120–122

Sweating, 123–124
with anxiety or depression, 3, 31

Swelling, 45, 125–126
in belly or abdomen, 26, 34, 55
in face, neck, or arms, 105

T

Tamoxifen, 114

Temperature. *See also* Fever
changes near death, 61

Testosterone, 114

Testicular prostheses, 89

Therapy. *See* Chemotherapy, Drug therapy, Immunotherapy, Radiation therapy

Therapy, psychological, 1, 2, 3, 28, 29, 30, 101

Thermometer, oral, need for, 44

Tiredness. *See* Fatigue

tlc, 50

Total Parenteral Nutrition, 134–135

Tracheostomy, 117–118, 119

Transplants, bone marrow, 16–17

Treatment. *See* Chemotherapy, Drug therapy, Immunotherapy, Radiation therapy

Trials, clinical, 21–22

Tube feedings, 131, 132, 135–136, 137

Tubes used in therapy, 131–132, 135–136

Treatment at home, 127–130

U

Ulcers
mouth, 71, 75–78
pressure, 109–111

United Ostomy Associations of America, Inc., 118

Urinary tract infection, 14

Urination
frequent, 15
lack of, 34, 47, 81, 126
near death, 62–63
painful, 14, 15

Urine, dark, 47, 81, 107

Urostomy, 117, 118, 119

V

Violent behavior and confusion, 25

Vision, blurred, 36, 38

Vomiting, 79–81
blood, 8, 10, 72, 81
and chemotherapy, 18, 19
and constipation, 26
and dehydration, 47, 79

Books Published by the American Cancer Society

Available everywhere books are sold and online at www.cancer.org/bookstore

CANCER INFORMATION

General

The Cancer Atlas (available in English, Spanish, French, Chinese)

Cancer: What Causes It, What Doesn't

The Tobacco Atlas, Second Edition (available in English, Spanish, French)

INFORMATION FOR PEOPLE WITH CANCER

Site-Specific

ACS's Complete Guide to Colorectal Cancer

ACS's Complete Guide to Prostate Cancer

Breast Cancer Clear & Simple: All Your Questions Answered

QuickFACTS™ Bone Metastasis

QuickFACTS™ Lung Cancer

QuickFACTS™ Prostate Cancer

> *Praise for QuickFACTS™ Lung Cancer:*
> *"The ACS has achieved its goal of providing overviews that tackle need-to-know issues and supply references for additional follow-up information as desired. Recommended."* —Library Journal

Symptoms and Side Effects

ACS's Guide to Pain Control, Revised Edition

Eating Well, Staying Well During and After Cancer

Lymphedema: Understanding and Managing Lymphedema After Cancer Treatment

SUPPORT FOR FAMILIES AND CAREGIVERS

Cancer in the Family: Helping Children Cope with a Parent's Illness

Caregiving: A Step-by-Step Resource for Caring for the Person with Cancer at Home, Revised Edition

Couples Confronting Cancer: Keeping Your Relationship Strong

Get Better! Communication Cards for Kids & Adults (bilingual communication cards)

Social Work in Oncology: Supporting Survivors, Families, and Caregivers

When the Focus Is on Care: Palliative Care and Cancer

HELP FOR CHILDREN

Because…Someone I Love Has Cancer: Kids' Activity Book (5 twist-up crayons included)

Mom and the Polka-Dot Boo-Boo

Our Dad Is Getting Better

Our Mom Has Cancer (available in hard cover and paperback)

Our Mom Is Getting Better

HEALTH BOOKS FOR CHILDREN

Healthy Air: A Read-Along Coloring & Activity Book (25 per pack; Tobacco avoidance)

Healthy Bodies: A Read-Along Coloring & Activity Book (25 per pack; Physical activity)

Healthy Food: A Read-Along Coloring & Activity Book (25 per pack; Nutrition)

Healthy Me: A Read-Along Coloring & Activity Book

Kids' First Cookbook: Delicious-Nutritious Treats to Make Yourself!

TOOLS FOR THE HEALTH CONSCIOUS

ACS's Healthy Eating Cookbook, Third Edition

Celebrate! Healthy Entertaining for Any Occasion

Good for You! Reducing Your Risk of Developing Cancer

The Great American Eat-Right Cookbook

Kicking Butts: Quit Smoking and Take Charge of Your Health

National Health Education Standards: Achieving Excellence, Second Edition (available in paperback and on CD-ROM)

INSPIRATIONAL SURVIVOR STORIES

Angels & Monsters: A child's eye view of cancer

Crossing Divides: A Couple's Story of Cancer, Hope, and Hiking Montana's Continental Divide

I Can Survive (Illustrated)*

*A Mom's Choice Awards® Finalist! (2007)